How to Lose Weight Without Working Out or Counting Calories

A Lifestyle Guide to Healthy Fat-Loss

By Radoslav Detchev

TABLE OF CON

ABOUT THE AUTHOR

Growing up, I didn't take care of my mind or my body. I wasn't strong, athletic, or charming by any means. I was addicted to video games and would play for 10+ hours a day. I had little emotional control and lacked social skills. Bowls of cereal, pizza, and McDonald's were staples in my diet while I survived on minimal sleep.

That all changed in 2013 when I started watching youtube videos showing the feats of strength a human body is capable of. Crazy acts of acrobatics and bodyweight strength inspired me to start training myself. At the time, I was attending school studying criminal justice but would soon transition into a Kinesiology degree to follow my passion.

Along the way, I found inspiration in the works of Ido Portal, Paul Chek, and Joel Seedman. These men offered incredible knowledge and a major paradigm shift away from what the mainstream media portrayed as health and fitness. The pursuit of movement over esthetics took over my training and with the help of the Chek Institute, my lifestyle started to become much more congruent with who and what I wanted to be.

After graduating with my Kinesiology degree, I went on to train Shaolin Kung Fu, Tai Chi, and QiGong in China for 9 months. Living in the mountains of Jilin province, I was able to dedicate myself to training my mind and body. Every day there was a challenge and an opportunity to improve. It is also where I started my online career as a content creator.

I drove across Canada from Vancouver and moved to Toronto after China to focus on helping people transform their lives. I refined my methods both inside and outside the gym to help serve my clients and the online audience. I've experimented on myself for over 10 years in order to see what works and what is straight up garbage.

While living in Toronto, I completed a Chinese medicine diploma program in order to add an energetic skill to my toolbox. This system focuses on getting to the root of the problem instead of just hiding symptoms. Through this, I learned that emotions are integral to health and the more equipped you are to handle them, the better your life will be.

I take a holistic and personalized approach to health. Training and nutrition are highly individual and everyone has to find out what works best for them. That's why I'm going to share with you the most important tools I've learned in order to help you.

It's time to get in tune with your body physically, mentally, emotionally and spiritually in order to listen and give it what it needs. This book is filled with the knowledge and wisdom that comes from over 13,000 hours of schooling, personal reading, coaching, and practicing.

Through my years of experience, the most valuable thing I can pass onto you is this. Your body has the final say as to what is healthy. If you don't look and feel good doing whatever diet and lifestyle plan you're doing, your body, state of mind, and emotions don't lie.

You can believe with all your heart that what you're doing is healthy, but intellectualizing and following a dogma when it's not working won't serve you. Do not become attached to a diet or habit that isn't producing health in your body just because you believe it should. This is when the mind takes over and tells the body what should be healthy. Listen to your body and let it show you what's healthy.

Science is never settled and will never be settled. That's why we have thousands of books, peer-reviewed papers, and experts on opposite ends of the spectrum yet still suffer from poor health in Western societies. Research will only take you so far. Real world results for your unique body is what you should be striving for.

Don't wait for some magic pill. Nothing will ever replace hard work and consistent effort towards your goals. Expecting something for nothing is a child's fantasy. If you do what is necessary and earn the results, you will be much happier and the results will stay.

HOW TO USE THIS BOOK

This book is filled with tools that will help you lose weight but the rate at which you lose weight will depend entirely on you. If you go on the extreme end of my recommendations, you could lose anywhere from 7-10lbs in the first week. I know, it sounds too good to be true, but I've personally done it myself as a lean individual.

When it comes to body transformations, this quote has always stuck with me, "A fence that goes up quick comes down quick". The faster you lose weight, the easier it is to rebound. It's best to have a gradual journey in the right direction. It's not about getting to your goal in 1 month vs 3 months. It's about maintaining or improving on it for years to come.

You will likely lose at least 5lbs in the first week if you follow just a moderate amount of the advice here. After that, aiming for 1-2lbs of fat loss per week will be attainable. Let's imagine you're 200lbs and want to reach 150lbs. A realistic timeframe for this would be 25-50 weeks at 1-2lbs/week. Is 6-12 months a reasonable amount of time for you to introduce new habits that can bring you a lifetime of health and fat loss?

Some of you might be disappointed with a 12-month timeframe. If you don't adjust and work towards your goals, the time will pass regardless. Where do you want it to be 12 months from now? Moving towards 150lbs or moving towards 250lbs? Set yourself in the right direction and don't worry about how long it takes.

It's better to start off doing the simple things that you can do. Don't force yourself to do things beyond your limitations. This is when the Yo-Yo snaps back, and you lose progress. You want to gradually build up the habits and become the person that deserves to lose the weight because you're doing what's necessary day in and day out

PART 1: YOU CAN LOSE WEIGHT

" The past doesn't equal your future unless you live there"
- Tony Robbins

I'm here to tell you that you can lose all the weight you want. You may not have succeeded in the past, but your past does not equal your future. It's time to leave any doubts and limiting beliefs behind. The reason you failed in the past is because you didn't have the right information and guidance.

Everything here has been tried and tested by yours truly. I know this works because I've done it and I've helped others do it too. I've experimented with weight loss and weight gain at extreme levels and that's where some of this wisdom comes from.

January 23, 2020. I was competing in a jiu-jitsu (martial arts) tournament, and I had to get to 135lbs to make my weight class. 7 days prior, I was sitting at 148lbs. I was able to drop 13lbs in a week while already being at 9% body fat. If it's possible for someone like me who doesn't have extra weight to lose, it's possible for you.

This was on the extreme side, and it wasn't sustainable for me nor did I want to maintain that weight loss because I was already so lean. However, if you're starting at a body fat of above 12% (where your abs are barely visible), you will be able to reduce your body fat levels and maintain them.

You can change the direction of your life if you focus on the present. Stop looking in the rear-view mirror of your life and start choosing where you want your future to be. Imagine your life 6 months from now. With your current habits, beliefs, and behaviors, will your body be more youthful, vibrant, and healthy? If the answer isn't a "Heck Yes!", it's time to take action.

Without activating these key fat-burning mechanisms you

will likely keep gaining weight, becoming sicker, having more body pain, and growing older will become inevitable. Take the next 6-12 months to transform your life and become the person you always wanted to become.

LOSING OVER 50LBS
DURING LOCKDOWN

This is my client and good friend Jen. She experienced first-hand what transforming her life looks like. I'm extremely proud of her and the progress she has made. With an integral part of her journey occurring during Covid-19 pandemic, with all the gyms closed, being stuck in her apartment and at the age of 44, Jen shows what any of you are capable of achieving.

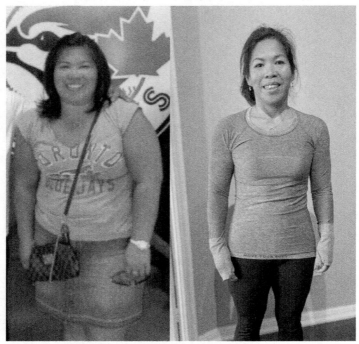

"Like many others, I knew how to dress for my shape and no one, not even myself could see what I was really hiding. I was content, not realizing I was fooling others and myself.

It had been a long time since I had stepped on a scale. I didn't want to face the reality of what it could say. One day, after weighing myself and seeing I'd somehow passed over 190lbs at a height of 5'2", I made the decision to invest in myself and get the help of a trainer.

Right before I was going to start training I ended up in a cast after falling and chipping my ankle bone! Perhaps I wasn't ready after all, was I really going to let another excuse get in the way of my health?

I pushed myself to train regardless of the injury because I didn't want to continue down the path I was on. I had made the decision to take my health seriously and make the necessary changes.

My journey started in 2015 and by 2018 I was down to 170lbs. I started to learn what I needed for myself physically but then took a pause to deal with some family matters.

I had plateaued and I'm sure due to some emotional and mental challenges I was undergoing with family matters, I fluctuated back up towards 180lbs until I started taking my health seriously with Rad in 2019. He started to help me to make changes outside of the gym.

He seemed to be happy and healthy so I decided to follow his advice. He never forced anything on me or told me that I "should" do something. I don't respond well when I'm being forced to do things in the drill sergeant manner.

He had an unorthodox approach from other trainers I'd been with and he would share the method behind his madness by explaining why he recommended what he did.

The way he explained things made sense. The more I did what he said, the better I felt and the more weight I lost. His theories brought tangible results. My favorite thing was that I didn't have to count calories or workout harder. I had already been working out without losing significant weight and was glad that "more training" wasn't the solution.

Rad was different, he opened my mind and brought awareness to other aspects of my wellness. Once I started paying attention to my mental, emotional and spiritual health and not just the workouts 3x a week which were not helping me lose weight anymore, things began to change dramatically.

It became clear to me that spending a few hours a week training was not going to counter my diet and lifestyle habits. Rad guided me through simple yet life changing concepts that I was able to apply gradually.

What you're about to learn is how I lost over 50lbs working with Rad. By the end of 2020 I was down to 140lbs. By 2021, I had dropped 19lbs to my lowest weight in over 25 years at 121lbs.

A large part of my results came from gradually changing my lifestyle. Making better food choices, beating bad habits, and all this during the height of the pandemic.

While I was watching other people put on weight from staying at home and dealing with the stress of everything, I was quietly chugging away and losing weight.

I still can't believe people's reaction when I go out with friends, family, and co-workers that haven't seen me in over a year. They don't even recognize me anymore.

What they can't see though is that it wasn't just my body that had changed. My mind and spirit were greatly impacted by the way I was living and I was able to see my relationship to food, emotions, and my body more clearly.

It is truly a lifestyle change that one must want to make for themselves. Losing 30lbs in a year may seem like a lot, but it can be done. I don't want to paint an unrealistic picture and tell you it was easy.

It's not easy to look into yourself and address all your weaknesses, shadows, and addictions but it sure is worth it.

There were struggles at times where I crept back up in weight, but all the tools that Rad shared helped me battle back. He has given me the wisdom and confidence to continue my journey and ensure I always know how to keep myself on the path.

Having read his book and gone down the journey myself, I know that anyone who wholeheartedly takes Rad's advice and puts it into action can see drastic results, not just with weight loss but in every avenue of their life."

The First 7 Days

Your first week of implementing my protocols will likely lead to a decent amount of weight loss. Losing anywhere from 5-10lbs would be reasonable. It would be unreasonable and unethical for me to tell you that all the weight you lose in the first week is pure fat, that's just not realistic without surgery. It is more realistic to lose 1-2lbs of fat in a week.

The majority of the weight you're going to lose in the first week is considered water weight. Due to a number of reasons (which you'll soon learn), people tend to hold onto a lot of excess water which can make you look puffy, swollen, bloated, have you feeling like you've got led in your body, and turn your fat-burning mode off.

This initial week will be exciting as we would all like to see results right away. This extra weight will be like a burden lifted off your shoulders that will motivate you to continue gradually losing more and more weight.

Alongside weight loss, these healthy habit changes will improve your energy, help you fight off disease, reduce body pain, increase your mood, regulate your emotions, and calm your mind. It's not just about losing weight, it's about feeling better too!

WHY YOU CAN'T GET RID OF YOUR STUBBORN FAT

There are 4 main reasons as to why you're holding onto so much water weight and why you look like it. Once you learn to control these factors, you'll not only lose water weight faster than a sack of potatoes being dropped off a building, you will also put your body into fat-burning mode.

1. Eating too many carbs (carbohydrates)

Carbs are 1 of the 3 macronutrient groups, the others being proteins and fats. When you eat 1 gram of carbohydrate, your body will store between 3-4g of water alongside it.

Carbs come in many forms and tend to make up a large portion of people's calories. Here are just a few basic foods that are largely carb based: bread, pizza, burgers, pasta, beans, legumes, quinoa, rice, power bars, bananas, berries, coca-cola, juice, coconut water and everything else with flour and sugar.

The dietary guidelines of those following a typical American diet is to have 45-65% of your calories come from carbs. If you're eating 2,000 calories a day, that comes out to approximately 225g-325g carbs. This equates to an extra 675g (1.5lbs) of water on the low end and 1300g (3lbs) of water on the high end. This is just from one day.

A 12oz can of coca-cola has 39g of sugar. That means just one can of coke can make you retain 117-156g of water weight. That's about 1/3 of a pound. Imagine if you're drinking 3 cans a day or even a 2L of soda. No wonder it's hard to lose weight.

One more thing to consider, eating 2,000 calories is the "average" amount in order to maintain weight. If you're consuming more than that, you're likely also adding fat along with that water as you watch the scale slowly creep upwards.

That's only one half of the story. Carbohydrates have another horrible effect that halts your body's ability to burn fat. More about that in the next section.

Now for some good news. This has been most of the calorie calculating we'll be doing in this book. As promised, your success will not be dependent on keeping track of calories or purposefully eating at a caloric deficit. What you eat and when you eat is more important than how much you eat.

2. Eating excess table salt

Sodium Chloride (NaCl), commonly known as table salt, is notorious for making people hold water weight. Table salt is an isolated substance that is simply not found in the wild and is used for its consistency and ability to be put into food without producing unwanted interactions. Reducing your standard table salt intake will help with weight loss.

In nature, we find things like sea salt and Himalayan salt. These salts can have up to 50 different minerals, creating a complex set of compounds that the body uses synergistically. When you isolate salt into pure sodium chloride, your body has a difficult time processing it, unlike its more natural brethren. Your body does not work well with isolated compounds.

Table salt, similar to carbs, will make your body hold excess water. It's not that salt is bad for you. On the contrary, salt has been vilified and the mainstream media would have you believe that you're better off never eating salt again. The reality is that you need salt. The problem is that table salt is in so many products that we are overloading ourselves with it.

Starting today, do your best to replace your table salt with a quality Himalayan or sea salt. Your body will gain much more nourishment due to the additional minerals which will help detoxification and fat-burning processes function better. Most processed foods contain table salt and a boat load of carbs. If you can reduce or eliminate these foods, you will not only lose water weight like crazy, you will tune up your body and activate your fat-burning mode.

3. High levels of inflammation

Inflammation is the process by which your body's immune system is activated to help fight off a virus or bacteria. However, sometimes your body may produce an auto-immune response where it attacks itself thus producing inflammation.

If you often experience joint pain (arthritis), muscle aches, fevers/chills, fatigue and even headaches, you could be suffering from chronic inflammation. When your body is chronically in attack mode, its energy and resources go towards that instead of towards healing, repairs, and trimming fat off your body.

Having chronic inflammation is like putting your body on constant high alert. It never gets a chance to rest and repair because it's always putting excess resources into defending itself. Inflammation can be thought of as a fire in the body. When your body is hot and on fire, what does it want? Water! Having excessive inflammation can cause your body to hold onto water in order to cool itself down.

Alongside making it difficult for you to lose weight, inflammation is involved in many diseases such as: cancer, arthritis, heart disease, asthma, and even Alzheimer's disease. By lowering your inflammation you will not only lose large amounts of weight but you're also increasing your overall quality of life.

4. Stress!

We all know stress is a killer, but it's also a water retainer, craving booster, and fat mongerer. The more stressed you are, the harder it becomes to stick to healthy habits and lose weight. When your body is in stress mode, it turns on innate survival mechanisms that force it to store as much fat and water as possible.

Imagine living on Earth 50,000 years ago. Stress could show up as a scarcity of food and water or during times of hunting or being hunted. When stress is triggered, it can react by sending the signal to store food and water because we're in danger of a famine happening and we might not get more resources soon. This causes cravings and pangs of hunger that are difficult to deal with.

Getting control over your hunger is pivotal if you want to lose weight. Having multiple ways to control stress and cravings is what will help you succeed in your journey. When you're calm and relaxed, you signal your body that it's ok to let go of some resources internally because there is plenty in the external environment. Your body doesn't know that there is a grocery store right next to you. It just knows the signal of stress.

Your body isn't meant to live in a state of chronic stress. Stress is extremely taxing on your body. 50,000 years ago, we didn't have email, texts, mortgages, 10 hour work days, and cell phones constantly sending a stress signal. We weren't living in a state of perpetual stress that our bodies are now battling daily.

Stress that came in the form of hunting or being hunted was a stimulus that did not occur on a 24 hour basis as it seems to for many people in modern society. Most likely, you would experience a stress response for a few minutes while you managed to escape.

During a stress response from an attack, your body releases cortisol and adrenaline into your bloodstream. When running, these hormones help increase the energy and strength in your muscles so you can escape. They signal to your body that it's a do-or-die moment and that everything must be diverted in order to survive.

All the resources from your body that were going to digestion, recovery, and repair are halted immediately as blood flow is redirected to your muscles. If you don't escape your attacker it won't matter if you digested your meal properly or repaired your tissues. You will be dead.

This is also why people tend to lose control of their bladder and bowels when under extreme stress. If you're running away from an attacker, you want to minimize the weight you're having to carry. The problem comes from your body's inability to distinguish a physical attacker from modern day stressors. It can't tell if a lion is chasing you or if it's just your boss calling you into their office. The stress response is the same.

Translate this to the modern desk jockey who sits in front of a computer for 8 hours a day, not to mention their leisure time. Constantly sending the signal to release stress hormones even though there is no direct danger. And since they're sitting at a desk, the hormones linger in their bloodstream for a much longer time as they're not being used up by the muscles.

With the stress mode engaged, blood flow and bodily resources are directed away from the digestive system, organs, and other tissues that are important for health. Without adequate nutrition along with removal of waste, these essential parts of your body are functioning far below their capabilities.

Before we dive deeper into exactly how you will be losing weight, it's important to understand why you would want to do the things presented here. Seeing the bigger picture will help keep you motivated and consistent. It's not about calories. It's about getting back in tune with nature in order to reduce stress and allow your body to heal itself.

TURNING ON FAT-BURNING MODE

The reason you have a hard time losing weight isn't because you're not counting calories. Your increased waistline is not so much a calorie problem, but something bigger and more preventable. Your weight gain (and loss) is due to two hormones: Insulin & Glucagon.

You've likely heard the word insulin before, however, you're about to learn why it's so important to your weight loss goals. Here's a quick and oversimplified explanation. Insulin is a hormone that regulates the metabolism of carbs, proteins, and fats by helping with the transportation of glucose into your muscles, liver, and fat cells.

Glucose is known as a monosaccharide. It is a type of carbohydrate that has been broken down to its most basic molecule. When you eat a piece of bread, your digestive system breaks the bread down into the smallest components possible so that the food can pass into your bloodstream and be transported around your body.

When you eat or drink calories, insulin is triggered in order to store those nutrients into your body. There are a few foods such as saturated fats and MCT oils that will produce a negligible amount of insulin, but for the most part, anything with calories will trigger insulin.

Insulin is an anabolic hormone meaning it's there to build up your body. It allows your body to store calories. Its main function is to help regulate blood sugar by not allowing it to be excessively elevated. If your blood sugar is elevated and insulin can't help reduce it, serious health problems occur, namely diabetes.

Realize that not all calories will trigger insulin equally. In general, liquids will increase insulin the most as they are absorbed much faster than solid foods. Eliminating liquid calories is an excellent way to stop insulin spikes.

Carbohydrates are the next fastest way to enter your bloodstream and trigger insulin. You may have heard of simple and complex carbs before. Simple carbs are easily broken down and tend to raise insulin much faster than complex carbs which take longer to break down. Think candy bars (simple) vs leafy greens (complex).

Next up, we have proteins which will elicit less of an insulin response compared to carbs. Finally, we have fats which tend to stimulate insulin much less as they take longer to break down and absorb. The faster a calorie can be absorbed and put into your bloodstream, the greater an insulin response your body will need to have. If the calories come from coca-cola, they will raise blood sugar levels quickly. If you eat 1lb of salad, it will take a much longer time for that to break down.

The glycemic index score of a food, which can be googled, will show you how quickly it is broken down into glucose thus giving you a gauge of how much insulin will need to be released to process it. The more insulin that is released, generally speaking, the more likely you are to store that food as fat.

There are two primary ways your body uses insulin to store energy. Short-term energy stores are known as glycogen. Simply put, glycogen is a collection of glucose (sugar) molecules that are readily available for the body to use. These are stored in your liver and muscle cells. Long-term energy stores are known as triglycerides, which are found in fat tissue.

If you want to lose weight, you need to prioritize accessing your longer-term energy stores of triglycerides. Learning how to do this is the primary focus of this book. Rather than utilizing short-term glycogen energy stores as your main source of fuel, you will be able to tap into your fat stores.

This is one of the reasons why counting calories isn't the main method used in this book. Because calories are not calories. If you eat 100g leafy green vegetables, the carbs, fats, and proteins in there will take a relatively long time to break down and enter your bloodstream. This triggers much less insulin compared to eating 100g of a candy bar that spikes your insulin way more.

Why Should You Care About All of This?

Depending on what you eat, it can take several hours after a meal to bring your insulin levels down to normal. When your insulin levels are elevated, it means your body is in energy (sugar and fat) storing mode. The secret to losing weight quickly is to reduce insulin. When insulin levels are elevated, not only do they cause you to gain weight, they also inhibit the function of glucagon which does the opposite of insulin.

Glucagon is the unsung hero of fat-loss. When glucagon enters your bloodstream to replace insulin, your body becomes catabolic by entering breakdown mode. With glucagon surging in your blood, fat-cells become stimulated to release their stores of calories into your bloodstream so you can maintain your energy levels. This is what I call Fat-Burning Mode.

When insulin is in the bloodstream, it inhibits glucagon because your body thinks there are plenty of calories available and coming in. There is no need to trigger the release of your fat-cell energy stores. Insulin suppresses access to energy stored in your fat cells.

Your body is being tricked into thinking there are calories when, in reality, they are gone. When you spike your insulin, glucose is stored away, which in turn drops your blood sugar levels below their resting norms. Now you start to feel the sugar crash. You are unable to access fat stores for energy because there is too much insulin in your blood.

This decrease in blood sugar, along with the inability to access fat stores, tricks your brain into thinking you're hungry because it has lower blood sugar compared to baseline. Thus, feeding the cycle of eating more food, spiking insulin, feeling low energy, and having to eat again.

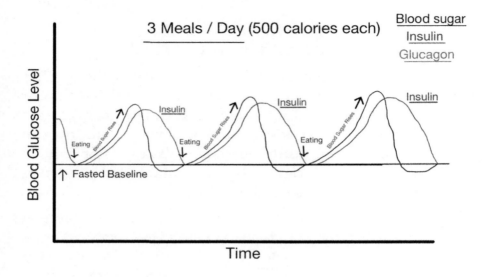

If you want to lose weight, counting calories isn't the secret. Instead, focus on reducing insulin and triggering glucagon release. It's about what and when you eat. In order to lose weight, you need to increase the amount of time glucagon is in your blood and reduce the amount of time insulin is.

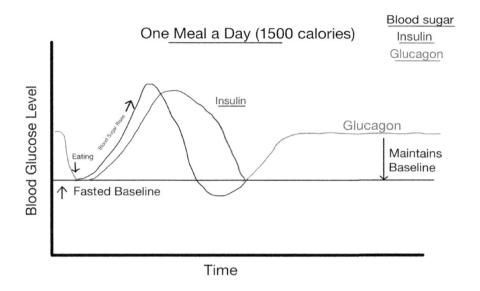

One Meal a Day (1500 calories)

Blood sugar
Insulin
Glucagon

Blood Glucose Level

Insulin

Glucagon

Eating

Blood Sugar Rises

Maintains
Baseline

↑ Fasted Baseline

Time

If you're a diabetic or even pre-diabetic, this book can help you improve your symptoms. You know your body and insulin requirements best. If you've been taking insulin for years, please don't just stop taking it. Consult your doctor, measure your levels, and get advice from your health care provider if you choose to adjust your insulin intake as you go along your weight loss journey.

You can go to https://radoslav.ca/FastingBenefits to see a video of me explaining this as well.

WHY I DON'T COUNT CALORIES

I'm not saying that counting calories doesn't work but it's never been an approach that I've personally stuck with nor used with clients. Let's be real, does anybody enjoy counting calories? If that was the secret sauce that makes weight loss work, why are there so many people who fail to maintain diets focused on calorie counting?

The hunger component, I would argue, is one of the main reasons people fail to comply. If your main strategy is to simply reduce your energy intake but you're not mitigating the effects of that on your hormones, you are fighting against yourself. For long term weight loss to work, the strategy you're using needs to be sustainable.

The traditional saying goes like this: "it's calories in versus calories out". As long as you reduce how much you're putting in and maintain or even increase your output, you will lose weight. On a basic level, the logic makes sense. When it comes to execution, I have a problem with the way most people go about solving this equation.

As you reduce your calories, your body starts to reduce its output. You need to give your body a reason to maintain a higher output than input. Unless you're using strategies to mitigate this (like the ones contained in this book), simply reducing calories without taking into consideration what you're eating and when you're eating will likely cause your metabolism to slow down.

That's why people who cut 500 calories out of their lives lose some weight, but then end up plateauing. Their metabolism slows down to match the input of calories. Not only that, but they tend to be more moody, fatigued, and drained from using up their willpower to not eat. The deliberate calorie cut tends to catch up with people.

Going from 2,000 calories of crappy food to 1,500 calories of crappy food is not the solution I advocate for. You can count calories if you wish to do so, but I'd rather see you prioritize the quality of the food you're eating and the time of day in which you eat it. These two factors, in my humble opinion, are more important than reducing your calorie intake.

Will your calorie intake decrease as a result of following my guidelines? There is a good chance of that happening, but again it's because you'll be focusing on eating better foods that satiate your hunger and give you real nutrition. It will also be easier because you will be manipulating your hormones to work for you, not against you.

Going Back to Your Roots

Bringing your body back to a state that's much more in tune with nature will help you lose weight and heal yourself. You may have heard of ancestral or primal living before, but perhaps you haven't so I'd like to share a little with you as to why everything you're about to learn is so powerful.

Everything in this book is geared towards moving you back in time. Simply put, our bodies have many mechanisms in place that rely on signals from nature to trigger it in order to be healthy. External stimulus plays an important role in DNA and gene-expression. Whether your body expresses genes for a certain disease or not is partially impacted by your lifestyle choices.

Our bodies have been evolving and adapting over the past 2,500,000 years to bring us to this very point in time. In the last 10,000 years or so, we have introduced technological advances that have pulled us away from the natural cycle of life. Many mechanisms in our bodies are chaotically thrown off by modern conveniences. Instant access to processed and calorie dense food, temperature controlled housing, a lack of movement, and a drastic increase in stress are just a few of the problems we must overcome.

Since weight loss is the primary goal of this book, we need to understand how your body views food. From an ancestral perspective, anytime we came across food, we would tend to eat as much of it as possible as we don't always know when our next meal would be. Your body is especially attracted to anything sweet in nature such as fruits which can provide an abundance of sugars to help fuel your body. And this is where the problems start in modern society.

Having 24/7 access to stupid amounts of sugary and processed foods is a problem. Your body hasn't adapted all that much in the past 10,000 years, let alone the past 100 years. Nowadays, you can take in such vast amounts of calories and your body doesn't know how to handle it. Its main option is to shuttle all that blood sugar into fat cells as fast as possible to avoid self-destruction.

The human body is very intelligent but it is often confused by living in the modern era. Because we were designed to live in nature, there are many smart things your body does that make a lot of sense to do in nature, but make little sense in the modern world.

Your body doesn't know that you can just go to a grocery store and all kinds of food is instantly available. Your body is an independent system that relies on itself to store resources in times of stress. It wants to eat high calorie foods and store fat when possible in order to safeguard itself.

It's time to start feeding yourself real food that will help control your cravings and your waistline. Get back in line with nature and discover the healing powers laying dormant within your body.

COMMIT TO YOURSELF

If you want to make a change, it's time to commit to yourself. Gone are the days of not being able to wear your old "Slim" clothes, having to buy new pants because your stomach doesn't fit in yours anymore, being embarrassed to take off your shirt at the beach, and getting out of breath from climbing a few stairs.

Today is the day where you change all of that. It's time for you to leave behind old limiting beliefs and behaviors that are holding you back in order to build true confidence in yourself. Just because you've spent 20, 30, 40, or 50+ years gaining weight doesn't mean you have to continue.

Through committing to yourself, you will build something that many people want but too few people have: Self confidence. And you're in luck because there is a simple formula for self-confidence. <u>Make commitments to yourself and then follow through.</u> That's how confidence is built.

Think of any relationship you've had. If that person said they would do something and they did it, your confidence in them grew. If they didn't do what they said they would do, your confidence decreases in them. Take this notion into the relationship you have with yourself.

Commit right now to changing your life over the coming 7 days. If you do exactly what I'm about to teach you, you will be so excited with the results that you will want to continue committing to yourself. You'll want to keep building confidence in yourself and soon enough, the people around you will also increase their confidence in you!

Belief in yourself is vital in this journey. Without belief, it will be hard for you to stick to anything. You will soon have a good understanding of why you're doing what you're doing and how it directly connects to your ability to lose weight.

If you have a spouse, family, parents, kids, roommates, etc., ask for their support. Show them what you're committed to changing so they don't pull you in a direction you don't want to go. It will also keep them from being offended when you turn down something that you would normally do with them.

Are you Ready?

If you feel ready, here are two tasks for you to do ASAP. Put this book down and come back after you have completed them.

1. Find an accountability partner.

Someone who also wants to lose weight and become healthier too. Look for someone who is willing to do the work like you and share this book with them. It's much more fun to share the journey with someone and have their support than to do it all alone.

2. Throw out all the bad food in your house.

If it's there, your mind will inevitably think about it. A lapse in willpower is much less damaging when you don't have the ammunition right there. Your journey will be much easier if cookies and chips aren't within arm's reach constantly. Battling against your environment is a lost war if you're just starting out your weight loss journey.

You may live with someone who doesn't want to throw out their bad food. In this case, you could ask them to hide it so it's not in the kitchen. If you believe in yourself and want to succeed, you know these two tasks will be very useful for you to complete as soon as possible.

Measuring Success

This is an important part of the process. Accept where your starting point is and decide never to come back here again. I've had clients that refuse to step on a scale and acknowledge how much they've let themselves go. I've even had clients start crying after seeing their weight. Don't underestimate how powerful this experience can be. Acknowledge where you are, maybe you're just 20lbs away from your target or 200lbs.

focus on becoming!

Measure your starting point and record it. When you hit the goal that you're happy with, I want you to be able to look back and see your journey. I highly recommend taking measurements and pictures. Snap a few selfies or get someone to help you take some pictures and videos. Less clothing is better. Make sure to get your front, side, and back. If you have a soft measuring tape, record your biceps, hips, waist, and thighs as well.

Now, measuring success by someone else's standards doesn't usually work. We agree that a scale is a simple, objective, and useful tool, but having more than just those numbers to look forward to can be helpful in keeping you motivated.

For you, successfully hitting your goal might mean fitting into your favorite dress or putting on your favorite suit again. Maybe you have a photo you love of yourself wearing that particular piece of clothing or even wearing no clothing at all. Put those clothes, pictures, or whatever it is that motivates you to lose weight out in front of you, on your nightstand, on your mirror, even on your TV if you must.

Remind yourself each morning why you're doing what you're doing is important to your success. When you can connect healthy habits with the destination of your goal, your mind will be much happier to go along for the journey. The more pleasurable you can make the experience, the more likely you are to follow through.

Having an overall weight goal you want to achieve is great, but keep in mind that it's not about the destination, it's about the journey. It's not just about losing weight, it's about who you become on the path to losing weight. You want the journey to be enjoyable and sustainable because it doesn't end once you hit your goal. You don't want to lose all that weight and gain it back, do you?

Focus on becoming rather than getting. Losing weight means gaining real skills in taking care of yourself, much like a mechanic takes care of a car. The discipline, self-confidence, and trust you create in yourself is worth the journey of becoming the best version of yourself. Looking at yourself in the mirror and being proud of yourself is success. The number on the scale is just a number. Be happy with who you see in the mirror.

The Truth about Diets

The food you eat matters. We know that eating real food is generally better for us compared to eating processed, synthetic, and denatured foods. Going back to the basics by eating what Mother Nature gave us is how you'll regain your health and lose weight.

There are thousands of experts with PhDs, peer-reviewed journals, and years of theoretical study of the human body, yet there still isn't a conclusive diet that everyone agrees on. People will continue to disagree with regards to what the best foods, diets, and exercises are for people to engage with until the end of time.

The problem is that although we all share many similarities, we also have many differences when it comes to our digestion and what's best for our unique body. This is largely due to your genes, DNA, lifestyle, and influences growing up. Before the past few hundred years, and especially the last 50 years, humans didn't have the ability to change their living location or have access to all kinds of food as readily as we do now.

Here's a simple example: Imagine someone with a family history that had lived in the hot climate of Mexico for thousands of generations moving to the cold weather of Northern Canada. The climate and the food available in that area would be greatly different and that person's response to those changes will likely have an impact on their health.

The truth is, our bodies were designed by nature to eat what was local and seasonal. Giving one specific diet that would serve everyone forever is not the approach I use nor is it realistic.

GUIDING PRINCIPLES FOR
EATING FOR WEIGHT LOSS

Here are a few simple rules that will give you a good foundation when it comes to diets and weight loss. The more you deviate from these, the more you move away from health and towards gaining more fat.

 1. Remove processed foods

If you're reading the label and don't understand what the ingredients are, you shouldn't be eating them. Avoid anything with sugar, high-fructose corn syrup, canola, soy or any vegetable oil variation. These oils are highly toxic to the body, increase inflammation, and will keep you fat.

2. Focus on real food.

Eat meats, vegetables, and fruits. Focus on foods that were available 10,000 years ago from Mother Nature. Don't confuse your body with fake foods that it doesn't know what to do with.

3. Eat until you're 80% full.

There is no need to stuff yourself. It makes digestion much harder, can make you feel tired, and will lead to over-eating. Tune into your body and don't overfeed yourself in one sitting.

4. Buy organic when possible.

Going to farmer's markets is a good option if you want to pay less and get local, in-season, and organic food. Having your food sprayed with a cocktail of chemicals that are meant to destroy lives will not help you get closer to health.

5. Enjoy what you're eating.

Do your best to season and put love into the food you eat. Eating food that you don't enjoy makes it harder for your body to digest and absorb the nutrients. It also makes it harder for you to adhere to good eating patterns.

We are all different

Although I give specific diet advice on foods to eat and foods to avoid, the best policy when it comes to diets (and anything else in life for that matter) is to try it and get feedback from your body. Maybe your body does well with eating beef but not chicken. Or you feel good with salads but not beans. Experiment and tune into your body. If a food is producing good results, keep eating it. If not, stop eating it.

When it comes to foods like quinoa and kale, the media will have us all believe that these superfoods will save the day. From personal experience, both of these foods destroy my intestines. Even though they are touted as amazing foods, my body doesn't handle them well.

There is no point in me blindly continuing to eat these foods while they produce this negative effect. For some of you, this might seem obvious, however, there was a period in my life where I was eating a decent amount of quinoa. I didn't recognize the damage it was causing me because my intellectual mind "decided" it was a healthy food and therefore I should eat it.

How do you know if a specific food is good for your body? The easiest way is to limit the amount of different foods you're consuming in a meal. If you have a 10+ ingredient meal, it will be hard to tell which food is causing you problems.

Signs & Symptoms of Food Problems

The best way to determine if what you're eating isn't working well is to be on the lookout for these key signs and symptoms during and after your meals.

1. You get a headache

2. You feel tired (or you take a nap)

3. Skin abnormalities (itching, redness, or rashes) on the face, tongue or lips.

4. Eyes become red, itchy, or burning

5. You generate mucus at the back of your throat

6. You start hiccuping (usually when you overeat)

7. Did you experience heartburn, nausea, or vomiting

8. Stomach distension and/or pain

9. Undigested food, blood, or mucus in your stool

10. Any other symptoms you might be dealing with that become exacerbated after eating.

When you eat food that enriches your body, you should have more energy after. You should feel vibrant, not like taking a nap. Pay more attention to your body and less attention to experts. It's good to research and learn, but your body is king and queen when it comes to the truth.

If a study shows that "X" food provided benefits to 80% of the people who consumed it, realize that you might be in the 20% that didn't get benefits and might have gotten a negative impact from it. Always rely on your body for feedback. If you look good, feel good, and are doing good, then chances are your diet and lifestyle are on point.

If you feel like something someone might step on in an off-leash dog park, then no matter how much science or data is backing up your theory, it isn't working and you should adjust your philosophy. Letting go of dogma and beliefs around health is an obstacle to acknowledge and work through.

You don't need to be perfect all the time. Perfection can weigh on you mentally and even has a medical term when you focus too much on eating healthy, known as orthorexia. If you eat and live well most of the time, you will see the results you want. If you only have a salad once a week and eat at McDonalds every other day, don't be surprised if you keep gaining weight.

Bridging the Gap

If you're trying to go from an unhealthy lifestyle to a healthy one, you will need to add new positive habits and remove old negative habits. In order to do that, some of you will be able to quit your old habits instantly (think smoking, drinking alcohol or eating McDonald's), however, the "quitting cold-turkey" approach will not work for some people.

Bridging the gap is how you're going to make these lifestyle changes as palatable as possible. At the end of each section, I will provide ways to modify my lifestyle suggestions to fit where you are in your journey.

For example, if you've never run a marathon, let alone 5km, you could try running a marathon everyday for 7 days. That probably wouldn't turn out well... Or, you could bridge the gap by committing to 3km a day for the first week. Then go 5km the second week and build on your successes in a sustainable way.

Some of you may already be somewhere on the spectrum of my recommendations so please pick the habit change that is appropriate for you. It wouldn't make sense for me to tell everyone to start running at 3km. Maybe you're already doing 10km a day and going down to 3km would be a step backwards.

Pick where you want to start on each habit and build from there. I would encourage you to do your absolute best during these first 7 days to help engrain the habits and to raise your level of motivation. When you look good and feel good, you tend to keep doing the things that get you there.

Do your best, even when you fail

I've failed many times. Diets, workouts, and lifestyle modifications have eluded me on my quest many times. It's been a long journey transforming myself from that boy who played video games all day and ate junk food. I had a lot of bad habits that have been shed and continue to work through my faults.

I have come far down my path and have helped others go through exactly what you're about to go through. I know that the things I'm sharing in the book work because they have changed my life and the lives of my clients. I also know that we can't be perfect everyday and accepting failure is important.

As committed as one can be, we all slip up. Don't take that as the end. Just because you had a cheat meal doesn't mean you need to quit and that you've failed. It's about getting back on the horse when you fall off. You've only failed when you choose not to continue improving your health.

THE PAIN TEACHER

The pain teacher is a metaphor I learned from Paul Chek. Pain in any aspect of your life is there to teach you something. The sooner you can see that the challenges you are facing are lessons to learn from, the faster you will grow as a person and the healthier you will become.

Physical, mental, emotional, or spiritual pain is a sign that you are not living in alignment with your highest purpose. We can all learn to listen to the pain in our life and what it's telling us. If you're sitting all day and your lower back is hurting, the pain is a signal to do something different. If you're gaining weight and it's taking a toll on you, that's a sign that what you're doing isn't working.

Imagine putting your hand on a hot stove. The pain mechanism is direct and immediate. You know that your hand is being burnt and thus remove it instantly. Most things that are burning you, metaphorically speaking, do not happen nearly as fast as a hot stove and therefore it makes it harder to distinguish what is causing the pain.

The steps you're about to learn for weight loss will also help you identify your pain teachers. Anything and anyone can be a teacher for you to get out of pain. Don't ignore the red-hot stoves in your life that are causing you to burn. Not just on the physical level, but on the mental, emotional, and spiritual ones as well.

If you keep doing the same thing, you're going to keep getting the same thing. Identify what isn't working in your life and make a plan to change. Most importantly, don't believe anything I say. What's written in this book isn't meant to be taken on blind faith. It's meant to give you an opportunity to learn about your body and how it functions.

"Intellectualism is a common cover up for fear of direct experience" - Carl Jung

Far too many people read books, watch videos, and get coaches but they don't apply what they learn. More knowledge isn't the answer. Activate and engage with what you read by having genuine curiosity and excitement as to how it will impact your life.

Knowledge will be useless to you unless you apply, test, and experience it for yourself. It's your job to convert knowledge into action, thereby making it wisdom. Knowledge doesn't impact the world until it's matched with hard work and application.

PART 2: REPROGRAMMING YOUR BRAIN

Your present choices create your future. What you eat today dictates your health in the future. The information you consume today creates your mindset in the future. Everything you do today has an impact on tomorrow in some shape or form.

Without intention, focus and active decisions you will always default to the easy way. What's easy today? Fast food, laying in bed all day, watching Netflix, not exercising, or consuming excess drugs and alcohol. It's not necessarily these things that cause problems but rather a lack of purpose and meaning behind their use.

The dose makes the poison and so the overconsumption of your vices will lead to negative health consequences and weight gain. Be honest with yourself: How's that been going for you up until now? If it's anything other than "Actually, very good", commit to taking small strategic action steps every day. To improve your life now and your future. Do not half-ass this.

Half-ass action will get you half-ass results. Half-ass results will suck out every bit of the motivation you have. If you don't see results, why would you want to keep pushing yourself out of your comfort zone? We are about to go deep into your foundations in order to help you lose weight and regain your health. Once you're healthy, you can go out and focus on everything else.

The Truth About Health

Health is not something you "just have". It's a skill you must learn. Losing weight is just like riding a bike or playing an instrument. It takes time to acquire the skill. Remember when you first tried to ride a bike. At one point it was a challenge for you. But with conscious practice you become better and better.

Riding a bike becomes easier and easier until you are so good at it that you consider it second nature.

The same principle applies to losing weight and living a healthy life. It starts with conscious effort to make the right decisions until it becomes second nature. Some got taught health skills from childhood while others didn't.

There's a concept known as Hebb's Law which states that "Neurons that fire together, wire together". Meaning that the more times you do something, the more likely you are to repeat that pattern, consciously or unconsciously.

Introducing new habits is like walking through a dense forest. At times your brain will want to take the beaten trails of the past. Old habits slip in and past behaviors rear their ugly heads. Building a new habit is all about repetition and traversing through the forest of neuronal pathways in your brain to create new habits and trails.

When you fall into old behaviors, you must be cautious and avoid the trap of beating yourself up. It's part of the process. You didn't give up on riding a bike because you fell down a few times did you? I don't think so. Don't give up on your health just because you get a few scrapes from falling along the way. Accept that you will slip up.

The exercises I have prepared for you in this section will assist you in changing your habits so you can lose weight and keep it off for good. Grab yourself a piece of paper, notebook, or journal before reading any further. There is little to gain if you read this section and go into the next without taking immediate action and writing down what I show you here.

Motivation

Motivation has likely failed you in the past when it came to weight loss. It fails most people because they start to implement healthy habits without first establishing why they want those habits and the benefits they are trying to achieve with them.

They have no real goals. Goals like: "I want to lose weight so I'll start eating a salad once a day" fail to motivate us because there is no emotional driver. No real reason to succeed in doing something new and uncomfortable.

You need to have deeper reasons and emotional connections to help carry you through these challenging times.

For example:

... I want to play with my children when they grow up.

... I want to be proud of who I am, how I look, and how I lead my family.

... I want to get out of pain so I can enjoy playing golf again.

People fail to lose weight due to a lack of clarity in their purpose and really defining why they want to succeed. I created 3 exercises to help you identify your purpose in order to build healthy habits and lose weight. Each exercise has multiple parts and will take around 10 - 15 minutes.

This is perhaps the most important part of this book and yet it has no direct application to weight loss in terms of methods to lose weight. However, without clearly establishing your motivation to succeed and how you're going to maintain it when things get tough you will likely fail to stay the course.

Take as much time as needed and have fun with these writing exercises. The more time invested here, the better your foundation for success will be. Setting the mood will really help stimulate your creativity. Being outside in nature will help as well. Get a cup of your favorite tea, remove your phone, turn off Netflix, and remove as much background noise as you can.

EXERCISE 1: IDENTIFY YOUR DESIRES

The Love List

Get a piece of paper/journal out. Don't do this on your phone, it will have a greater impact if you write it down on a physical piece of paper that you can put on your fridge, nightstand, bathroom mirror (any high traffic area).

Answer these 3 prompts:

- What do you love to do?

- What makes you happy?

- What makes you excited to get up in the morning?

Don't limit yourself here. Maybe there is something you've only done once in your life or have never done and might not see that as a "realistic" option. That doesn't matter, write it down if it makes you happy and excited!

If you have a hard time identifying what you love, you can flip the question in reverse. What don't you love? What gives you nightmares? What stops you from jumping out of bed in the morning? What is it about your life that you don't enjoy doing/being/seeing? After you create this list, you can write the opposite of each one to convert the nightmares and move towards love.

The Health List

With your love list complete, you are now going to make a few additions.

Answer these 2 prompts:

- Things I know are healthy and I'm already doing

- Things I think are healthy and I'm willing to do

Do your best to make this list knowing that as you continue to read this book, you will be adding to the list of healthy things you're doing and are willing to do.

Recognize that when you do these things that help you lose weight and make you healthier, you are giving yourself love. You may not enjoy certain actions (yet), but you will soon have a process to transform your mind and body into enjoying things that are healthy yet are currently uncomfortable and foreign to you.

The Healthy Love List

Now that you have a concrete list of things you love (or nightmares reversed) along with a list of things you believe to be healthy, put that list somewhere that is highly visible as a reminder (fridge, bathroom mirror, desk etc).

Reaching your weight and health goals mean you'll be able to do more of what you love. If there are things on that list you haven't been able to do because of the shape you are in, let the vision of yourself engaging in the action motivate you.

Do as many of these healthy love items as you can each day! They will improve your mood and motivate you to take care of yourself. As you become healthier you open up new possibilities. More opportunities to explore come into your life because you now have the clarity to bring them in and the energy to pursue them.

The really important part about this is to acknowledge and say in your mind that through doing this action, you are giving yourself love. This is a crucial part of the process of instilling a new healthy habit. Our bodies and minds are often disconnected from what feels good in the moment and what is good for us in the long-run. By doing this, you're helping condition your mind to crave the things on your love list.

Let's say one of your healthy love items is going for a walk. As you're walking, consciously acknowledge and say to yourself "by walking, you are giving yourself love". This is pivotal for re-programming your brain and for you to fully step into the healthy love items you've listed for yourself.

Another example would be eating a healthy meal. As you eat your meal, acknowledge that through eating this meal, you are giving yourself love. Visualize all the benefits that come along with eating your healthy meal and hold those thoughts with a positive energy around the activity.

Why is it so important to do this? Let's take a look at the opposite side and where a lot of people make the mistake. We know that exercising, walking, playing a sport, eating a healthy meal or even just going to bed on time is good for us, but we often tell ourselves the opposite in terms of mental talk.

Imagine if you will, a scenario where you decide to start working out to improve your health. Each time you go to the gym, do you hype yourself up about how much love you're giving yourself and how much you're going to benefit from it? Or does this run through your mind: "I don't want to sweat, I don't know what I'm doing, I feel awkward, this hurts, why am I here, I think I'll skip today, or I'm gonna be sore after"?

What about when you choose to have a healthy meal? Are you eating that salad thinking about how much love you're giving yourself and how you're improving your health? Or are you cursing having to eat your veggies while wishing you were snacking on a candy bar?

If you think something sucks but you're doing it anyway just to "be healthy", you're going to have a hard time maintaining that behavior because you are associating negative things instead of positive things while doing the healthy habit.

The reason you wrote the list of things you love is to be able to remind yourself that you understand how this is beneficial for you and that any act of kindness towards yourself shouldn't be met with resistance from the mind, but rather should be invited.

Your mind can make things easy, or it can make them hard. You decide. Once you understand this and truly start to live it, you no longer need motivation to do the things that are good for you. You start doing them automatically because your mind and body are in agreement instead of fighting each other through sheer will-power.

Now that you've stated to yourself what healthy love is for you and have safe ways to give yourself love, realize that being healthy and taking care of yourself will allow you to love yourself more. You'll be able to do the activities on your healthy love-list more often and with more presence and purpose.

This exercise and practice is so crucial that without it, anything else you try to do for your health will likely fail. This is the fuel that keeps good habits going even when you don't necessarily feel like it. Without the experience of love, it's hard to wake up in the morning and do the things you should do to be healthy.

If you can add the habit of acknowledging when you are giving yourself love, it will give you an incredibly strong foundation to build any other habit or lifestyle change.

<u>Caveat</u>

At this point, you might be saying to yourself, "But Rad, some of the things I love doing aren't healthy for me". That's cool and 100% normal.

You have two options:

1. Dig deeper into understanding what you are getting from that action and see if you can replace the underlying feeling/satisfaction you get from it with something else.

- Going to a night club and getting drunk might be replaced with joining a social club around one of your hobbies.

2. Accept that it is detrimental and that you are willing to take other actions to compensate for it.

- You enjoy partying on the weekends and don't want to give it up. Good news, you don't have to. You can make up for it by doing other healthy activities during the week in order to balance out the partying.

The reality is that not everything we love doing will be healthy for us. As long as you are making a conscious choice and taking responsibility for your actions, you are living a life of mindfulness and presence. You don't have to live like a monk.

EXERCISE 2: GOAL SETTING

We will now integrate your healthy love list into your goals. Most of us are familiar with outcome goals, however, process goals are my favorite when it comes to self-improvement.

Outcome goal: something to be reached.

Fit into my clothes from 5 years ago, lose 20lbs, have $10,000 in the bank, live abroad, or find a significant other.

Process goal: based on doing a task. Think of this as a habit.

For example: Eat 5 servings of vegetables everyday, drink 500ml of water upon waking, do one thing a day for a client that gives them value beyond expectation, go into nature on Sundays, do 100 push ups daily, or talk to a new person every day.

An outcome goal can take days, weeks, months, or years to fulfill whereas a process goal is about taking action each day in order to move closer to the desired outcome.

Process goals can have positive self-talk and love attached to them. Eating a salad can be a process goal you choose to engage with and as stated before, you can create positive emotions when eating salad by engaging in positive self talk.

Outcome Goals

Write down at least 3 outcome goals for each of these 6 areas of your life: Physical, Mental, Emotional, Spiritual, Relationships, & Career

You can reflect on your healthy love list for inspiration and use it to help create your goals.

Examples

- Physical: I love doing Jiu Jitsu, therefore, a physical outcome goal for me would be to get my black belt in Jiu Jitsu.

- Mental: I love studying languages, therefore, a mental outcome goal for me would be to speak French comfortably.

Keep this list in a visible place so you're reminded daily of what your goals are (fridge, bathroom mirror, desk, etc.). You might be saying to yourself *"but Rad, I just want to lose weight, what do goals in my career, relationships, etc. have to do with that"*?

Everything in your life is connected. The clearer you become with these goals, the easier it will be to stick through your weight loss journey so that you can live out your life goals. Perhaps your career goals require you to have lots of energy, vitality, cognitive clarity, and creativity. It's hard to achieve that when you're not in a healthy state.

Maybe you want to meet the man or woman of your dreams. If you can have a healthy relationship with your mind and body, do you think it will help lead to a healthy relationship with another person? The more excitement you can generate with goals in different fields, the more motivation you will have to succeed.

Process Goals

The next step is to convert each one of your outcome goals into process goals that you can do each and every day.

From the previous example, it would look like this:

1. I love doing Jiu Jitsu, therefore, a physical outcome goal for me would be to get my black belt in Jiu Jitsu

- Process goals for this would be: to go to 3 Jiu Jitsu classes a week, watch 1 technique video a day, write what I learned into a journal after each class, stretch for 5 minutes each day, or stretch after Jiu Jitsu class.

2. Mental: I love studying languages, therefore, a mental outcome goal for me would be to speak French comfortably.

- Process goals for this would be: Read 5 minutes of French each day, review french flashcards for 5 minutes each day, watch a French movie once a week, or learn 5 new French words each day.

Once you've done this, pick just one process goal from each category that you think is the easiest and doesn't take a lot of time or effort. Start simple and easy using the lowest commitment process goals. If you're at a loss for process goals, fear not. That's where the rest of this book comes in handy. You are about to be armed with a shiny new toolbox of habits that you can use to lose weight and regain your health.

Process goals don't have to be big. They can even be things you already do, this will help you become even more consistent in the aspects of life which you are already good at. As the weeks and months go by you can gradually add more process goals or increase your commitment to the current ones. The important part is to make it as seamless and easy as possible in the beginning by not taking on too much.

It may be unrealistic for you to spend 4 hours a day completing your process goals if you've never spent 20 minutes dedicating yourself to your goals. The lower the bar for entry, the greater your chance of success. When you're working towards your process goals, acknowledge that through doing the action, you're giving yourself love. Allow yourself to fully experience that feeling. When you do this, you're teaching your body to associate feel-good hormones with an activity that is good for you.

Just like a dog that receives a treat (love) after doing a trick, so too will your brain and body come to realize it's receiving a treat each time you engage in a process goal. Soon, it will start craving those good feelings through your positive habits and life becomes much easier because you don't have to rely on willpower and motivation.

EXERCISE 3: RE-PROGRAMMING

Now that you have your goals and healthy love list laid out, the final step in the process is to re-wire your brain. This is where so many people go wrong when they set new habits and goals for themselves, especially when it comes to weight loss.

They only do this process once! BIG MISTAKE!

Realize that when you wake up tomorrow morning, you may not want to engage with what you have just laid out. This is due to old-patterns, habits, behaviors, and emotions coming through. Years and years of conditioning and programming your mind doesn't go away overnight. Just like a dog that's spent its whole life peeing in a certain spot can't be expected to change overnight and pee in a new area just because you told it one time.

Repetition is the mother of all skills.

Imagine your subconscious mind as a completely separate entity, much like a dog or a child. If you praise and acknowledge good behavior and re-state what the good behavior is, they are more likely to behave that way. By repeatedly affirming to yourself the things you love doing and the process goals you want to engage in, you will train your subconscious mind to be drawn towards those things.

Affirmations can be one of the most powerful tools you use to re-wire your brain into doing things that are beneficial for you. However, many people don't do it properly. It's not just about being clear on what you want, it's about stating everyday what you're willing to do in order to achieve your goal.

Making the connection with your conscious and subconscious mind between your goals and the process is crucial. When you combine the acknowledgement of love, this becomes a triple threat combo that will greatly increase your chance of success.

Affirmations

If you've already completed the previous two exercises and practices, then you're ready to begin combining your healthy love list, outcome goals, and process goals into a script that you read every morning.

Taking from the previous example, I can affirm that I am a black belt in Jiu Jitsu over and over again, but that will never happen if I don't put the work in. So, a better approach is to state what I'm willing to do in order to achieve this.

I'm working towards becoming a black belt in Jiu Jitsu by:

- Going to class 3x/week

- Watching 1 technique video each day

- Stretching everyday

- Competing 3x/year.

Use these prompts to help you create your own script. Change the words to suit you:

- I _____ through _____

- I am _____ because I _____

- I will _____ by _____

- I am becoming _____ since I _____

- I will achieve _____ because I _____

- I will be _____ because I _____

Examples:

- I give love to myself everyday through my self-care routines.

- I am more calm and peaceful because I meditate for 5 minutes every morning.

- I will lose 20lbs by eating unprocessed foods, exercising 4x/week, and drinking only water.

- I am becoming a better partner since I spend 20 minutes each day reading a book on communications and relationships.

- <u>I will achieve</u> a black belt in jujitsu <u>because I</u> train 3x/week, watch 1 tutorial every day, and make notes on what I learn.

- <u>I will be</u> the best version of myself today <u>because I</u> actively choose the beliefs I want to program into my mind and read my affirmations every morning.

A few suggestions

When it comes to the mental, emotional, spiritual, and relationship categories, you can make immediate shifts. For example, if you're someone who struggles with anger issues, you can say something like:

"I am calm and am able to catch anger rising inside me and tame it before it comes into the physical plane because: I spend 5 minutes everyday meditating, I read books on anger control, I watch videos and do exercises to manage my temper."

When it comes to physical and material things or career, don't lie to yourself. If you're 300lbs and stating that you're 150lbs, you and your subconscious recognize that as false and it will not reprogram you. If you have

$500 in your bank, repeating to yourself that you have $1,000,000 isn't going to help you.

Instead, focus on affirming your outcome goals by stating the process goals you're willing to do to achieve it.

"I will weigh 150lbs because I eat unprocessed food, drink only water, exercise 4x/week, and go to bed by 10pm."

In the beginning, your scripts should be short and simple. I am listing many examples above. A more realistic script if you're just starting out is:

"I will weigh 150lbs because I only drink water".

If you are currently drinking 2L of coca-cola each day, switching to just drinking water could be a giant leap for you but you know the results will be worth it. Keep it simple. Once drinking water becomes second nature, then you can modify it to something like this:

"I will weigh 150lbs because I only drink water and eat a dairy-free diet".

Gradually add to and modify your affirmations. Start simple and easy. Make the modifications impactful but limit the time, energy, and money commitment in the beginning. What I'm suggesting is the equivalent of waking up one morning and saying either:

1. I'm going to run 1km everyday for a month

Vs

2. I'm going to run a marathon everyday for a month

Option 1 may take 15 minutes on the first day but can come down to 5 minutes once you acclimatize.

Option 2 will likely take you 6-8 hours the first day and you might be so sore you won't run for another week. Which one has a great chance of succeeding in the long term and building your foundation?

Using positive present tense is also ideal for programming your mind. Don't use negatives like – I don't smoke, I don't eat bad food, I never stay up late. Instead, use the positive form: I love myself more than I enjoy smoking, I eat healthy food, I go to bed by 10pm.

With these exercises and practices, don't feel glued to anything on the list. If something doesn't provide love to you anymore, remove it from the list. If your goals change, update your list. As you grow and evolve, it's likely that your passions and love will too. Listen to your heart and adjust.

This practice is best done in the morning as soon as you wake up. By reading these affirmations ASAP, you're priming your brain to look for opportunities in the day to achieve these actions. Leave your scripts and lists close to your bed or in the bathroom so that when you wake up, you have quick and easy access to these.

As you read these affirmations, you can visualize yourself doing the process goal needed to achieve the outcome goal. If you can see yourself in your mind's eye completing the task, you are reinforcing the habit before you even do it.

Now that you've completed all the exercises, the final thing left to do is to execute! Commit to making yourself better day by day through these simple practices.

PART 3: THE HABITS

These habits are the foundations to your success. Read through and start to gradually incorporate them into your life. If you successfully build on these, your health and your weight will improve. Imagine your health as a pyramid. The bigger your base is, the higher your health can go. If you try to do too many highly specific things without a strong foundation, the results will be poor. I'm talking about expensive surgeries, supplements, pills, and crash diets to name a few.

Don't complicate things. Do what you can. Each section offers many options for lifestyle changes. You do not need to do all of them at once. Pick the easiest ones and build your foundations. Avoid starting 20 new habits. You're better off adding 1-3 easy modifications per week and easing yourself into long term and sustainable habits.

#1 DRINK WATER

"The cure for anything is salt water: sweat, tears or the sea."
- Isak Dinesen

I hated drinking water for a large portion of my life. Milk was my go-to liquid of choice. It was a running joke in my family that I would go to a restaurant and order milk as an adult. Once I started discovering just how important drinking clean water is for the body, I did my best to switch over.

Switching was a struggle as I found the taste of water to be bland at best and nasty at worst. What I didn't realize is that not all water is created equally. If you're drinking tap or bottled water, you're getting a lot of extra particles in there that you can't see with your eyes but your taste buds and your body definitely feel.

When Jen was in the midst of her weight loss journey, she was drinking filtered water from her fridge. I decided to try it and could immediately taste the plastic particles from the hoses. I invited her to a 30 day experiment where she would switch her filtered water for mine.

She wasn't convinced that there would be a difference but she was willing to try nonetheless. She started by using something called a Berky which uses carbon filters to clean water through gravity. After a few weeks, she tried her fridge water again and could taste a big difference. Once you're used to drinking clean water, it's hard to go back.

After the experiment, Jen was sold on the difference in water quality. She felt better and was continuing to lose weight. Jen went on to get a 6 stage reverse osmosis water filter with remineralization installed in her kitchen. She finds it hard now when she travels to get the same level of quality water.

Quality Counts

Water is a critical component of your fat loss plan; one that is often overlooked. You want to make sure you are drinking enough water, but also the right kind of water. Avoid tap water as much as you can. It contains chemical cleaners such as fluoride and chlorine that cause harm to your body. These chemicals kill bacteria and will mess up your gut bacteria, similar to what an antibiotic would do.

Tap water often contains recycled water from the city sewage system. This water has medications that people have taken, processed, and then excreted down the toilet. These medications are difficult to remove with a simple Brita filter. Realize that you could be drinking water that contains birth control, blood pressure medication, and who knows what else. Don't drink straight distilled water either. Pure water, without minerals, cannot be used by your body because it cannot conduct electricity.

When distilled water enters your body, it starts extracting minerals from your bones in order to make itself useable. This is even worse when the water is acidic, like most bottled water and tap water. If you can, buy a water filtration system like a Berkey or install something in your place. There may even be natural springs in your area where you can refill containers for free.

Adding a pinch of Himalayan or Celtic Sea salt to your water will help mineralize it. This will make it easier for your body to absorb and use the water. Don't over do it and make your water taste like salt. A small amount will do the job and it should not make it taste salty. When possible, drink mineral water that has at least 300 ppm total dissolved solids. This can sometimes be found on the labels of bottled water if you have to buy it.

You Gotta Drink The Stuff

10 Billion Billion (yes, I wrote billions twice on purpose) biochemical reactions every second require water to take

happen When you're dehydrated, these biochemical pathways become slow, inefficient, and create a huge problem in your system. Chronic dehydration can contribute to long-standing health problems. By choosing to drink water, you will experience many health benefits.

Imagine a car that has only half of the oil it needs to properly lubricate the engine. Is that car going to last long, maintain its horsepower, or get good mileage on fuel? I doubt it. Let's imagine again that that car has no oil left to do anything. All the parts in the engine start rubbing together, creating friction and heat that wears down the system and renders it broken.

Your body is much smarter and more adaptable than a car but the same principle applies. You need water to lubricate your body and keep all systems running well. You need to put the right fluids and fuel into your body for it to function properly. Unlike a car engine, your body has the ability to partition where water goes.

When you allow yourself to become dehydrated, you force your body into having to choose which pathways to prioritize. If you're low on water, chances are that your muscles and joints will be the first to have their rations taken away. No wonder so many people experience joint and muscle pain.

Good hydration will also help you age slower. Much like your muscles and joints become dry and dehydrated, when skin becomes dehydrated it tends to wrinkle, shrivel, and dry out. If you want to look and feel younger, look no further than the original fountain of youth.

Reduce Insulin

Making this change alone can transform your life dramatically. This is one of the easiest and fastest ways to lose weight and improve your health. Sounds too simple, doesn't it? When we factor in everything you've just learned about inflammation and insulin, you'll see how this one tip alone can help you shed crazy amounts of weight in a short period of time.

When you drink anything with calories, you create an insulin response to some degree. If you're drinking a can of coke, juice, or even coconut water you're creating an insulin spike and pulling your body into fat storing mode. There are a few borderline exceptions like bone broth that does stimulate a tiny bit of insulin but provide so many benefits that it can be worth it.

Be aware that diet soda drinks, which may have no calories, can also cause an insulin response. The sweetness from the artificial flavors tricks your brain into thinking that sugar is coming into the system and your body preemptively releases insulin. Likewise, chewing sweet gum may signal your body to prepare for incoming calories.

Remember that liquids absorb into your bloodstream much faster than solid food. The faster it goes in you, the faster your blood sugar goes up, the more you're triggering a greater insulin response. Therefore, you're staying in sugar and fat storing mode for a longer duration because it will take more time for your insulin levels to come back down.

At this point, you might be thinking to yourself:

"Wait a minute, I thought you wanted us to lose water weight. Doesn't drinking more water add to my water weight?"

Not really. When you don't drink enough water, your body does everything it can to hold onto what it has. When you drink more water, the body takes in that fresh water, rehydrates itself, and gives the signal to release old water along with anything else the body doesn't need. This aids in the detox process as well.

Don't worry about putting on water and weight from drinking more water. Remember, it is those 4 main factors mentioned earlier that cause the majority of water retention. Carbs, salts, inflammation, and stress are your biggest enemies. The more water you have in your system, the more equipped your body will be to fight off those 4 factors.

How Much Water Should You Drink?

As a baseline, drinking half your body weight in ounces is recommended. Using a body weight of 200lbs, you would need a minimum of 100 ounces of water each day. If you're using the metric system, you can take your bodyweight in kilograms and multiply it by 0.03. This will give you the liters per day. A 100kg person would need at least 3 liters of quality water per day.

Equations aside, the main way to see if you're hydrated enough is through the color of your urine. If it's pale light yellow you're good to go. If you find yourself going to the bathroom multiple times in an hour, chances are you're overdoing it by drinking too much water in a short period of time. If it's dark yellow, you're probably dehydrated.

Bridge the Gap

1. Drink clean water by avoiding tap and plastic bottled water. If possible, make the investment by buying a quality water filter. Spending money on clean water is a bigger priority than spending money on supplements. If you must, Evian is your best choice of water when traveling. When you read the label on a water bottle, you want to see at least 300 ppm (parts per million) of salt.

2. Commit to drinking 1 cup of water before drinking whatever you're craving. Your cravings are just your body's desire to rehydrate. It is rare that someone is suffering from a coca-cola deficiency and must drink it. I used to drink 2-3L a day of milk. I craved it as my go-to thirst quencher. When I realized it wasn't doing my body any good, I kicked the habit by using this technique.

It made me realize that I was just thirsty and my craving for milk eventually went away. This strategy only works if you commit. There can be no wavering when you feel the urge to drink something else. In the beginning, you may drink the water and still decide to have whatever drink you want. And that's cool. Eventually, your body will remember that it's craving hydration, not a can of coke or a coffee.

1. Drink 1-2 cups (250ml-500ml) first thing in the morning. Prepare a water bottle or glass so that when you wake up, it's immediately available. Add a tea-spoon of organic apple cider vinegar or a spritz of lemon if you want a boost in digestion. Drink this through a straw to protect your teeth.

2. If you for some reason don't like the taste of regular water, you can start with drinking carbonated water. You can also add sliced cucumber to it for some extra taste. In the long-run, I don't recommend getting most of your water from that source but it can be a way to ease yourself into drinking more water.

3. Commit to drinking only water before, after, or during a certain time. For example, until 2pm, you only drink water. Or after 10am, you can only drink water. Or, while you're at work (9-5), you only drink water.

4. Buy a bottle (1-2L) for your water. Commit to drinking 1-2 bottles of it during your day.

5. Avoid drinking too much water in the evening. I suggest getting most of your water intake during the day as you don't want to interrupt your sleep by having to wake up during the night to go to the washroom.

What About Coffee?

Although coffee has been shown to potentially have a positive effect on fasting and aiding fat loss, I personally don't recommend it. Certain drinks, like coffee, will dehydrate you. If you're trying to add more water and hydrate yourself, it doesn't make sense to drink something that's counter-productive to that goal like coffee.

The main reason I don't recommend drinking coffee is because it's tricking your body into thinking it has energy when it doesn't. When you feel tired, the secret isn't to stimulate your body with endogenous substances. The secret is to give it rest, good nutrition, and less stress.

Coffee gives you an artificial boost of energy. This kind of chronic stimulation depletes your body of its resources and drains you. What you really need is to boost the vitality of your body so you no longer require coffee for energy and instead run on your body's natural fuel.

Another downside to coffee is that if you drink it too late, it can have a negative effect on your sleep. The average half-life of coffee in humans is about 5 hours. Meaning that after 5 hours, half of the caffeine you consumed has been used up. However, this is just average. Some people have a half life as short as 1.5 hours for coffee while others have a 9.5 hour half life.

One final note on coffee and all products that are heavily researched and marketed: it's a multi-billion dollar industry. Consumers in the USA alone spent $74 billion in 2015. Science and research can be skewed to show positive results which can be why you see so many articles coming out on the benefits of coffee. With such a massive industry and so many people invested and hooked on this drug, people want to believe it's good for them.

Companies that spend millions of dollars to produce research don't want to find out that their product is having a negative effect on people. If a corporation funds a study that finds less than favorable results, there is no one forcing them to publish and release the study. They can, therefore, run a study as many times as they want and change variables, populations, etc. until they produce a study that shows what they want.

This is why I always say that you shouldn't trust what anyone says, even me. Do your research and then experiment in order to see how your unique body reacts. Coffee may be beneficial for some and detrimental for others. When you get to the root of it, are you drinking coffee as a crutch or do you just have it as a treat once in a while?

I want to be clear as I'm sure the coffee enthusiasts won't be too happy with me about this one. It's not necessary to give up coffee to lose weight, or be healthy. If the reasons listed above resonate with you, I would encourage you to reduce or eliminate your coffee intake. If you need coffee to get through your day but eventually want to quit drinking it, here's how you can start.

Bridge the Gap for Coffee:

1. Stop drinking it after 12pm as it can cause poor sleep if it's consumed too late.

2. Avoid Starbucks, Tim Hortons, or any mainstream franchised coffee sellers. Since they have to make their products with a consistent taste no matter where you are in the world, they have to process and preserve their coffee a lot in order to stabilize and standardize it.

3. Buy ethically-sourced, environmentally-friendly and organic products from local coffee shops.

4. Only buy black coffee or espresso (without sugar or milk) to reduce calories and to not trigger insulin production in your body.

5. Make your own coffee (without sugar or milk).

6. Buy organic beans and grind them yourself. Pre-ground coffee tends to be a good environment for mold to grow in. You don't want to consume mold on a regular basis.

7. Switch to organic teas like dandelion root tea or dandyblend.

8. Eliminate the need for caffeine from your life because your lifestyle grants you abundant energy.

#2 START FASTING

"Instead of looking outside of ourselves and counting potential enemies, fasting summons us to turn our glance inward, and to take the measure of our greatest challenge: the self, the ego, in our own eyes and as others see us."

- Tariq Ramadan

While I was training Shaolin Kung Fu in China, I ate some questionable meat that caused me severe digestive distress. This crippled me during training and day to day life. I dealt with it mostly in silence due to embarrassment. When I came back to Canada, the symptoms kept getting worse and worse.

After seeing a doctor, finding blood in my stool samples and even getting a colonoscopy (where they stick a camera up my butt), I was diagnosed with IBS (irritable bowel syndrome). Without going into gross detail of what I was suffering through, here are just a few symptoms I experienced: going to the bathroom 10+ times a day, gas, bloating, cramping, undigested food and diarrhea.

If I had a decent bowel movement once a month it was a cause for celebration. The IBS was particularly brutal when I had to train 5 clients in a row and was excusing myself in brief moments on the hour when I transitioned from one person to another. This was a horrible way to live, and something had to be done.

Fasting literally saved my gut and quality of life. After doing many extended fasts for 2-3 days, my gut started healing itself. I became more aware and in tune with what caused me intestinal distress. Through improved food choices, fasting, and emotional awareness, I've been able to overcome my diagnosis of IBS. If you're suffering with any digestive issues, giving your system a break from food might be the best thing you've ever done.

The Magic Bullet

Fasting is the closest thing to a magic pill that I know when it comes to losing weight and improving overall health. I've personally experienced its healing ability and have had clients achieve great success using just this tool alone. There are many ways to practice fasting and this section will cover the best ways for you to start doing it. Once you realize how much more powerful fasting is compared to counting calories, you'll see exactly how you can lose all the weight you want!

Fasting is when you go for an extended period of time without taking in calories. To be clear, fasting doesn't just have to be about eating and consuming calories. It can also be applied to other things such as cell phones, Netflix, or even smoking. The idea is that you refrain from taking in calories (solid or liquid) by designating times of the day to eating/drinking. This is what gives you the power to reduce insulin and stimulate glucagon.

Remember, when you take in calories, especially carbs, you increase the amount of insulin in your blood. When you fast, you are triggering the release of glucagon which in turn stimulates your fat cells to be metabolized to access the stored energy inside. The longer you fast, the greater the effects of glucagon become. The longer you go without food, the more your body has to break down its own fat cells to provide you with the energy you need.

In order to access your body's energy stores, you need to understand the 3 main locations where glycogen (sugars) and triglycerides (fat) hide. When you eat, insulin helps your body put the calories in your muscles, liver, and fat cells. It tends to be stored in that order as well.

The liver and muscles hold glycogen, which is a form of short-term energy storage that can be accessed quickly. Your fat tissue holds triglycerides, which are a form of long-term energy storage. Muscles store energy for themselves. When you

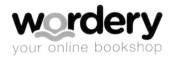

"If you only read the books that everyone else is reading, you can only think what everyone else is thinking."

Haruki Murakami
Norwegian Wood

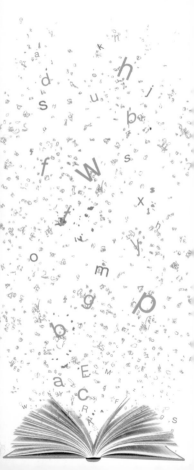

wordery

your online bookshop

use a particular muscle, you are using the glycogen that's stored inside it. If you workout and do bicep curls, you are using up the stored energy in the biceps.

The liver works as a bank of energy for the entire body. About 100g glycogen can be stored in the liver. These calories are slowly released into the bloodstream as needed. Engaging in fasting helps to empty the liver. It takes anywhere from 8-12 hours for liver glycogen to become depleted. Once this occurs, the body starts producing more glucagon in order to access the energy in fat cells.

When your muscle and liver stores are depleted and you eat, the body uses insulin to send the calories there first. This short-term storage of energy is easily accessible compared to the long-term storage of fat. If your liver and muscle cells are full, excess calories are sent to your fat cells. When the liver becomes depleted, your body starts devouring its own fat cells for energy because the bank of quick-access energy has run out.

The manipulation of insulin and glucagon is far more crucial than the amount of calories you eat when it comes to losing weight. Through fasting you can lose weight even while eating the same amount or even more food in a day than you normally would.

Counting Calories vs Fasting

We hear the word "calorie" all the time, but what is it? Calories are a unit of measurement for energy. A single calorie is equal to the amount of energy needed to raise the temperature of 1g of water by 1 degree celsius. If you're scratching your head wondering what raising the temperature of water has to do with you gaining or losing weight, welcome to the club.

Counting calories is an oversimplified model that's used to market products to you and to give you a rough idea of how much energy one food will provide vs another. There are 3 macronutrients that provide you with calories. These are proteins, carbohydrates, and fats.

1 gram of protein = 4 calories

1 gram of carbohydrate = 4 calories

1 gram of fat = 9 calories

When you look at this in isolation, you might think that fat will make you fat because it provides double the energy compared to the other two. However, eating fat doesn't necessarily make you fat and you'll see in the next section why.

Isn't a calorie a calorie? If you eat 2000 calories, does it matter what the food source was? Will any combination of carbs, proteins or fats that equal 2000 calories have the same impact? A calorie is not a calorie due to the hormonal impact. If you eat 2000 calories of chocolate, pasta, and coca-cola vs veggies and meat, do you think there would be a difference?

Absolutely! Chocolate, pasta, and Coca-Cola will spike your insulin much higher compared to veggies and meat. It's also much easier to eat a large quantity of processed foods vs nutrient dense veggies and meat. This is because real food satisfies your cravings while fake food does not.

Not only that, the veggies and meat are providing you with much more nutrition because they have a complex of vitamins and minerals whereas the processed sugary foods don't. Here's the beauty of fasting. Whether you're ready to change your diet or not, fasting will help you lose weight. Fasting works with any diet, but there are of course more ideal foods to eat when your goal is weight loss.

You may have heard the old adage of eating every 2 hours to keep your metabolism up. This simply isn't true and will have the opposite effect if you're trying to lose weight due to the constant insulin activation. Let's say you're using the traditional counting calories approach. You've done the math and now know that eating approximately 2,000 calories a day would allow you to maintain your weight.

You cut your calories by 500 in an effort to lose weight by choosing to eat 1500 calories a day. Since there are about 3500 calories in one pound of fat, it should take you 7 days (7x500 calories) to lose 1 pound. In the beginning, this may work, but if you're not fasting, you're actually working against yourself in the long run.

If you're not fasting, you will inevitably end up slowing down your metabolism. If you're eating breakfast, lunch, dinner and snacking in between, you're constantly raising your insulin levels. Overly elevated insulin levels lead to a reduction in accessible energy in your bloodstream.

Even though you're eating less calories, your body is having a hard time accessing your fat stores for energy due to the insulin. In order to lose weight according to the calorie counting model, your output of calories needs to be greater than your input of calories.

But if your body can't access its fat stores due to insulin, you're relying mostly on your daily input of calories to fuel your output. Instead of your body running off 2,000 calories, it has to do the same functions (moving, eating, working, etc.) with fewer calories.

This eventually causes a decrease in your energy and a decrease in your metabolism as your body starts to reduce its output to match the input of 1,500 calories. This is the opposite of what you want. At this point, because you're eating all day, your body is reliant on the quick-access energy of sugar and carbs instead of being able to reach down into its own fat reserves for energy.

You're inadvertently slowing down your metabolism to match 1,500 calories because you can't access the fat stores due to insulin from eating all day. If you've tried to lose weight in the past, you've likely hit this wall without understanding why it's happening. Keeping your body in a state of elevated insulin levels while decreasing your food intake is a surefire way to agitate your emotions, induce cravings, and ensure that you don't maintain the weight you lost.

Let's imagine instead that you decide to start fasting this week by doing an OMAD (One Meal A Day) style protocol for the next 7 days. In this scenario, you're eating one meal a day, and therefore having 7 meals during your week. You're only elevating your insulin 7 times during the entire week.

In contrast, if you're living like a typical person by eating breakfast, lunch, dinner and snacking in between, you could easily elevate your insulin levels 7 times in one day! I don't care how many calories you cut; you will have a hard time losing weight like this.

If you were to eat as many calories as you could in one meal, you likely wouldn't hit 1,500 calories, let alone 2,000 calories. You would have one spike of insulin and then have 23 hours to recover from it. Since your main goal is weight loss, I also wouldn't recommend trying to stuff yourself to hit those calories. Eat until you're satiated and no more than 80% capacity.

Here is how to safely and realistically start incorporating fasting into your lifestyle. If you have or are already fasting, this will show you how to increase the results you can get.

Flexible Fasting

There is a major caveat before we move forward with this section's bridge and protocols. Fasting is a tool! When it comes to fasting, there is a time and place for each of these methods. If you want to lose crazy amounts of weight, doing the protocols near the end will get you there.

That being said, the goal shouldn't be to stay there. Once you've hit a weight you like, you can back off and do more sustainable fasting. It isn't realistic to do 5 day fasts every week for the rest of your life, but you may want to do a few of them on your journey to losing weight. Once you've lost the weight, doing 16 hours of fasting a day is more realistic and sustainable.

If you feel as though you're re-gaining weight at any point, such as after a vacation, you can increase the intensity of the fasting again to lose the pounds you gained and then come back to a normal routine. Remember, in order to maximize access to fat cells for their energy, which leads to weight loss, you need these 3 things:

1) Depletion of liver glycogen (8-12 hours)

2) Reduction of insulin (No calorie intake)

3) Increase in glucagon (Access your fat cells easily)

Beyond Fat Loss

Many people use food to regulate their emotions. It's important for you to understand that in the beginning, you're going against your body's wishes and patterns. There will be resistance, but that's ok because it's an opportunity for growth. Instead of using food to fill a void or uncomfortable feeling, you now have the option to focus on the void and see what you're really missing.

Although you may have bought this book to lose weight, losing weight is not about going from 200lbs down to 150lbs. It's about who you become in order to do that. Without the process of "becoming", you will not be able to maintain the weight loss. Think of people who have liposuction only to regain the weight because they didn't make a change and become someone different.

Another example would be lottery winners. 70% of lottery winners end up going broke and a third of them declare bankruptcy. That's right, 33% of lottery winners go bankrupt! Why? Because they didn't become the person who has millions of dollars by learning to earn. They won the money and had no idea how to manage it.

Having a goal is important, but it's not just about achieving the goal. It's about who you have to become in order to achieve it. Losing weight is great but it's only a physical representation of what you had to overcome mentally, emotionally, and spiritually. Truly going through the journey of losing weight shows who you have become.

If you shortcut the process of becoming by using liposuction, lottery tickets, magic pills etc., you only cheat yourself from the growth you could have experienced. Don't rob yourself of the opportunity to build discipline, work-ethic, emotional control, self-confidence, self-respect, and so much more.

I had a deeply profound and spiritual message come to me during a fast. I used to struggle with fasting in the evenings because I was craving popcorn and chips. My body wanted salty comfort foods at night after a long and stressful day.

During what I would describe as the biggest craving I've had in my entire life, which occurred about 30 hours into a fast, I was able to focus inwardly and see what was really going on. As ridiculous as this may sound, I was truly suffering from this craving at that moment. I was having withdrawal symptoms from food and my body was not happy.

As I focused inwardly on this state, I could see the neurons in my brain that were asking for salty chips and popcorn. By choosing not to relieve myself from the hunger pains through distracting myself, I saw what they were asking for. They wanted <u>love</u>, not salt.

As a child and through adulthood, when those neurons were asking for love, I had been confusing the signal by providing chips and popcorn. Instead of recognizing what I truly needed, I had been filling a void and numbing myself to what my body was asking for.

This paradigm shift was a breakthrough for me and my clients, and hopefully for you too. Are you substituting love with emotional eating? I invite you to explore negative feelings, emotions, and voids as you journey through fasting. We will go into more detail on how you can go about doing this in a later section.

Put that Cookie Down!

This one tip has saved my fasts countless times. Commit to waiting 5 minutes when a craving hits. You may feel the immediate need to eat what you're craving but this will pass. Sit with that feeling and explore it instead of trying to fill the void with food.

Chances are, you're not actually hungry. If you have weight to lose, then you have the calories on you (stored as fat) to support yourself and you're not snacking because you're hungry, you're snacking because of old patterns and habits. If you wouldn't dive into a pile of broccoli and carrots, you're probably not starving. You're learning how to deal with the emotions and food addictions that have been leading you down a path you didn't consciously choose to go down.

Learning to make your fasts more manageable is what will allow long term compliance. Understand that you will likely get some fasting symptoms in the beginning if you're not used to it. This is normal and will improve.

It's normal for you to experience these symptoms:

1. Hunger
2. Headaches
3. Irritability
4. Fatigue
5. Trouble Sleeping
6. Constipation

These go away within a few days or weeks and are replaced with abundant energy, clear thoughts, and improved digestive function. When a craving hits, use this to help reprogram the cells in your body that are asking for your comfort food. This is what I did to overcome eating popcorn and chips at night.

As you feel the craving come on, commit to taking 3 deep breaths and saying, "I love myself". Additionally, you can drink a glass of water to help rehydrate yourself. It may take more than 3 breaths to calm your body down but with practice, this method will reprogram old habits. It will help change your state of being and ultimately lose weight because you overcame the mental and emotional drive to eat when you didn't need to.

Another way to make your fasts more manageable is to start by replacing meals with bone broth. Bone broth is healing for the digestive system, and it contains a lot of goodies that will make your joints and skin feel much better. Bone broth also carries a heartiness to it that very few other liquids can match. Although it does have a little bit of calories, it won't impact your fasting that much and is a better alternative than eating.

Drinking carbonated water is also a good option when you feel like eating something. The bubbles help to fill your stomach with gas, which expands it and helps signal to the brain that you're not empty. If you are working out and fasting for more than 24 hours, reduce intense exercise that isn't strength focused. Doing CrossFit or high output sports will drain you and amplify your cravings.

It's especially important when you're fasting to add a little bit of Himalayan, Celtic, or sea salt to your water. If you're not getting enough salt in your diet because you're fasting, you may feel weak and dizzy from a loss of salt. These salts, also known as electrolytes, will help balance out your body and provide important functions throughout the body. Naturally, you sweat and excrete these salts and without food to replenish them, things won't work as well.

Following the guidelines of all the sections in this book will greatly impact your cravings and ability to stick to a fasting protocol. The next step will be especially helpful in reducing your hunger.

Bridge the Gap

1) Only drink water. This stops insulin spikes from drinking calorie laden liquids during and between meals.

2) Stop Snacking. Keep your current main meals (breakfast, lunch, dinner) but remove snacks.

3) Don't eat your first meal until a specific time. When you wake up in the morning, avoid taking in calories until a time that you decide upon. Let's say you choose not to eat until 10am. Combining this step with the next step is how you're going to gradually work into what's known as an eating window.

4) Don't eat after a specific time. Set a time for yourself after which you will not consume anymore calories. 6pm is a great time to stop eating as food digestion tends to slow down at night. You don't want your body to be focusing on digesting while you're sleeping. You want it to focus on repairs (more about this in the sleep section). If, however, your family eats at 7pm and it's a valuable social time for you, don't sweat the extra hour, enjoy the benefits of seeing your family.

5) The 16-8 eating window. This is what most people mean when they use the term Intermittent Fasting. 16+8=24 hours in a day. You fast for 16 hours and eat for 8 hours. The choice of when you eat is up to you. As suggested earlier, starting at 10am and finishing by 6pm will give you an 8-hour window during the day. This is the ideal time as it's not too close to bedtime and it's only a few hours after you wake up. The bulk of the fast happens while you sleep which makes it much easier.

6) The 20-4 eating window. This is also known as the warrior diet and will give you a few extra hours in fat-burning mode. Fast for 20 hours and eat for 4 hours. You can get about 2 meals during this window. Again, if your intention

is to lose weight, this eating window is not about fitting in as much food as you can in order to make it to the next day. Eat in moderation and eat later in the day so that you're not starving while trying to sleep.

7) OMAD. Eating one meal a day adds another level of intensity to your fasts. If you do, I highly suggest eating later in the day, sometime in the afternoon or beyond. It's easier to stay hungry for a few more hours instead of eating breakfast, getting hungry at 5pm and going to bed wanting to eat.

Do you remember the beginning of this book, where I told you that I dropped 13lbs in 7 days? This was the fasting method I used. Alongside that, the only food intake I had was 1-2 cans of tuna for my one meal. I don't recommend eating that small amount of food for a long duration. In the next section, you're going to understand why I chose tuna and why it worked so well when done with OMAD fasting.

8) 24-48 hours fast once a week. Designate 1-2 days a week that you can fully commit to fasting. For example, your final dinner is Sunday night at 5pm. You won't eat again until at least Monday 5pm, but you could also set yourself to not eat until Tuesday 10am or anytime up to 5pm. Being consistent with this practice and combining it with 16-8 will give you great success.

9) 48 hours fast. The deeper into the fast you go, the more weight you will lose because your body is running purely off of your own stores of fat. This is the perfect sweet spot for most people who want to lose a lot of weight. It's like OMAD, but every other day. Once you eat your meal, wait two days before you eat again. When you fast this long, people tend to think they will lose muscle mass, however, you're actually saving muscle mass compared to eating multiple meals and cutting calories.

Since your body has easy access to energy from fat, it limits the amount of muscle breakdown that occurs. Your body also increases its human growth hormone release by up to 1,200% in order to help preserve your muscle. When you eat multiple times a day, this doesn't happen. When you restrict calories but keep your insulin levels high, the body can start breaking down protein in the muscles to provide energy. Naturally, it prefers to use its excess stored fat to provide energy. The body doesn't want to break down useful muscle when it has a legitimate store of energy in fat cells.

10) 72+ hour fasts. The longer you stay in a fasted state, the greater the effect. The first 8-12 hours of fasting yields the least benefits because your body still has carbs coming from the liver and some insulin in the blood. As you push further into fasting, each hour becomes more valuable compared to earlier hours in terms of fat-burning.

Your body also starts going into what's known as autophagy. Auto = self, phagy = eat. This self-eating state is important for your body as it gives it the opportunity to destroy old and damaged cells in order to stimulate the growth of newer and more powerful cells. Because your body isn't anabolic while you're fasting, it doesn't have new material coming in to maintain the usual processes. Weak cells end up dying, leaving you with stronger cells.

It's like running a broom and vacuuming through your body, cleaning out the old and leaving the strongest cells. If you decide to do these prolonged fasts, limit physical activity as you don't want to add extra taxation on your body. You also want to be careful coming off of any fast that is beyond 48 hours as your digestion has shut down. A heavy meal afterwards can be harmful. You should focus on slowly introducing foods such as bone broths, stews, and soups for the first day or two. Gradually build up to soft foods. What I'm saying is… do not have a turkey dinner after a 5 day fast!

#3 CUT CARBS

"Dear Stomach, you're bored, not hungry. So shut up"

- Anonymous

When I was in university, I spent about 2 months trying to put on as much weight as I could. Essentially, I was doing the exact opposite of what I'm suggesting you do here. On top of packing meals for myself, I ate fast food between classes to get as many calories as I could.

My two biggest commitments and methods for gaining weight were to measure out and eat a 1,000 calorie block of cheese along with drinking a minimum of 2 liters of apple juice every day. Back in 2014, I was studying the effects of insulin in my human physiology class and figured that I should do everything in my power to keep my insulin elevated all day.

The main way I achieved this was by drinking apple juice all day. The problems came about a month into my experiment. I found out the negative effects of constantly elevated insulin levels. As soon as I put anything into my mouth, I would start getting massive headaches.

I did manage to put on weight but the headaches became so unbearable that I thankfully stopped the ridiculous diet. A few weeks later, I went to the dentist and found out that I had 6 cavities! Force feeding myself processed carbs and mainlining sugar into my veins was a firsthand experience of insulin overload.

If you're overdoing the fast food and soda pop but don't feel these effects, that's normal. When your body has to deal with that level of toxicity, it numbs itself to the pain in order to function. Drinking sugar all day was a shock to my system that was so different from my everyday norms I was able to notice its impacts.

Many people don't realize just how bad they feel because of years of damage and adaptation. Once you clean up your lifestyle, you will be able to feel the effects of fake processed foods when you choose to indulge in them. Your taste buds will also change as you make healthier food choices. Going from oversaturation to natural flavors might seem like a hard transition, but once you're on the other side of a clean pallet, you'll realize just how unnecessary sugar is in most foods.

Know Your Enemy

Carbohydrates are the enemy of anyone trying to lose weight. Carbs will stimulate more insulin than proteins or fats and thus have the highest potential to keep you in Fat-Storing mode. Carbs will also cause you to hold a lot of extra water. You'll be shocked by how your body and mind change when you cut down on carbs for a week. You'll feel lighter both physically and mentally.

If fat-loss is your biggest goal, you should reduce carbs until you hit a satisfactory weight. I don't want you to eliminate carbs forever. I don't think you want to either. I just want you to be conscious of their effects and decide when they're appropriate in your diet.

As you become better and better at fasting and reducing your carbs, your body will adapt to using fat as its primary fuel source. Your body loves to run off of carbs (quick energy) if you're eating a standard American diet and aren't adapted to burn fat (long-term energy). Once you turn on fat-burning mode, cravings will go away and you'll be fueling your body primarily with the fat on your body.

Carbs and Fasting

Cutting carbs makes it easier to fast as focusing on proteins and fats will keep insulin levels lower, giving your body an easier time regulating your energy and cravings. They will also tend to take longer to break down and will keep your appetite down.

The faster you can get into a state of low insulin, the easier it's going to be for you to reduce cravings and not be tempted to eat early. Remember, high levels of insulin in your blood forces your body to remove the sugar (energy) from your blood and push it into your fat cells.

This drop in blood sugar levels signals your brain that there is a lack of accessible energy on board. This triggers you to want to eat. The more you keep your blood sugar at a balanced level, the less cravings you will experience. When your body doesn't go into panic mode because it can access the energy stored in your fat, you have a much easier time sticking to your routine.

The Keto Craze

The keto diet is a prime example of the carb reduction strategy. When you stop eating carbs altogether and focus on eating primarily fat, your body starts to produce something known as ketones at a much faster rate. Ketones are the byproduct of broken down fat cells that provide you with energy. A true keto diet will have you getting upwards of 90% of your calories from fat.

Eating pure fat isn't very appetizing to me and likely isn't to you either. Many people think they are engaging in a keto diet when they eliminate carbs, but in order to achieve this state where ketones are abundant and your primary source of fuel, you need to really reduce your protein intake to 5-10% as well.

Although there is a time and a place for this type of diet, I don't generally recommend this. Protein is important for your body. You can achieve a similar result without force feeding yourself coconut oil every day. By reducing your carb intake and focusing on prolonged fasting, you can stimulate ketones.

Extended fasting will get you into what's known as ketosis once your body starts adapting to it. Ketosis is when your body is burning significant amounts of fat for energy because it has run out of carbohydrates to fuel your body.

When ketones become abundant excess amounts start to become detectable. You can test your ketones by buying ketone strips and urinating on them if you're interested in an objective measure of your fasting and diet modifications. The higher your ketone readings are, the more accelerated your fat-burning is.

Not All Carbs Are Created Equally

Let's get clear on what I mean by carbs and which ones you should be removing. Technically, vegetables and fruits are carbs, but I don't encourage you to stop eating them all together. I'm suggesting you remove the processed, simple and high glycemic index carbs.

Vegetables are a complex form of carbohydrates and take a much longer time to break down and enter your bloodstream compared to a simple carb like white rice or bread. Therefore, the amount of insulin produced will be significantly lower. Another benefit to vegetables is that they provide fiber and nutrition that helps you feel satiated. This is key in fighting off hunger cravings.

Getting a large amount of calories from vegetables is difficult. If you based your diet on veggies alone, it would be hard to eat 2000 calories due to the sheer volume of food you'd have to eat. The more you can fill yourself up with nutritious food that your body can process, the less cravings you will have and the more your food will support your health.

Raw vegetables tend to be harder to digest. If you have any issues with vegetables or have weak digestion in general, I highly recommend cooking or steaming your vegetables. It may destroy some of the nutrients, but, if it improves your ability to digest and absorb them, it is worth the effort to cook them.

Fruits

Fruits are another source of carbs that I'd consider beneficial, however, you may want to limit your intake depending on your goals. Fruits contain much more sugar compared to vegetables.

They have natural sugars which are better than processed ones like high-fructose corn syrup, but they are sugar nonetheless.

If you want to have fruits, I'd suggest being conscious of their insulin raising effects and limiting your intake. When you eat them in their full form, the fiber inside helps slow down the absorption of the sugar. I don't want to demonize fruits, I just don't want you eating 5 sweet potatoes, 4 apples, 7 bananas, and 4 avocados in one sitting. Having one is ok, but having an excess amount will not help you lose weight.

Although they can contain a lot of nutrition, it's especially important to be wary of smoothies and particularly juices as the fiber has been stripped away or broken down meaning that they will raise your insulin much more than their solid form counterparts. Getting fiber from vegetables and fruits is important.

Experiment

Eating food should be like running an experiment. When you eat, do your best to be present and aware so that you notice if the food is helping or hindering you. Most likely you will already know which foods aren't good for you, but perhaps there is a food that you eat often and are unaware of its impact.

If you experience negative symptoms while eating a specific vegetable, fruit, fat, or protein, try to reduce or eliminate that food. Some vegetables and fruits tend to cause people problems due to naturally occurring chemicals that purposefully interfere with our digestive system.

Contrary to popular belief, most plants don't want to be eaten. They want to thrive, grow, and spread their seeds. Unlike animals that have legs and can escape their predators through movement, plants are rooted to their location. For protection, they produce chemicals that disrupt our digestion. That's why many plants in nature are not edible to us. They've created their defense through chemical warfare so we don't eat them.

This goes beyond the scope of this book, but if I've piqued your interest, I highly suggest reading "The Plant Paradox" by Steven Gundry and "The Carnivore Code" by Paul Saladino.

These 2 books do a good job explaining why you may want to avoid certain fruits, vegetables, and legumes and what you can do if you want to enjoy them without suffering the consequences. When someone has a peanut allergy, the symptoms can range from mild to deadly. Much like that, we all have certain intolerances to food that need to be avoided.

For example, I can't digest raw or even cooked vegetables well so I limit my intake. Also, eating foods like quinoa, lentils and beans don't do my body good. They cause me to become bloated, gassy, and often don't digest well. Pay attention to your body and find the foods that serve you best.

What's the Best Diet?

As I state throughout this entire book, there is no "best diet" because we're all different. I've provided suggestions that have worked for myself and my clients. Try them out for yourself and see how you feel. Your ancestry, DNA, genes, upbringing, stress levels, and years of eating certain foods come together to create a version of you that has unique dietary needs.

With all that said, here is a list of foods that are low in carbs and high in nutrition. Test out these foods and see which one's can be staples in your weight loss diet.

1) Free-Range Eggs

2) Wild Fish

3) Grass-Fed Beef

4) Organic Pork

5) Grass-Fed Lamb

6) Organic Chicken

7) Wild Game Meat

Above ground vegetables:

1) Carrots

2) Celery

3) Leaks

4) Asparagus

5) Onions

6) Garlic

7) Mushrooms

8) Leafy Greens

There are many more vegetables you could eat but I've chosen the ones that tend to work well with most people. If you do have digest issues, I recommend checking out the FODMAP diet. Experiment with the foods they allow and don't allow to help improve your digestion.

This is a list of fruits and berries that contain more carbs. You can limit their intake to the degree that you see them impacting your weight loss. A handful of blueberries is ok. An entire basket or carton will impact your insulin levels.

1) Blueberries

2) Strawberries

3) Raspberries

4) Blackberries

5) Apples

6) Bananas

7) Watermelons

8) Honeydews

9) Mangos

Cheat Meals

Some people can quit anything cold turkey and transform their life in a moment. The rest of us mortals, myself included, will need some time to adapt. It's ok to schedule cheat meals if you need them. Recognize your starting place and work to improve from there. If you're currently eating fast food 2 times a day, 7 days a week, cutting that down to 1 time per day is a 50% improvement.

You will get amazing results if you can stop eating most carbs starting today, but if you don't think that's realistic, do your best and gradually move towards reducing them. If you can give it 100% for a week, I recommend trying. The more processed foods and carbs you keep in your diet, the more cravings you will experience. I've learned this lesson many times in my life. If you eliminate bad foods, you stop craving them after a few days.

When you do have your old foods again, your cravings will return. If you decide to schedule a cheat meal or your willpower breaks down, limit the damage. The less bad food you eat when you cheat, the easier it will be to bounce back into fasting and Fat-Burning mode. If you would normally eat a full candy bar, eat only half of it and throw the other half out.

If you find yourself in the midst of a craving and are satisfied with it, throw out what's remaining. You don't have to keep eating it! But hey, maybe you were brought up to not waste food. Why would you throw it out? Because it's not food! Candy bars, chips, ice cream etc. are not real food. They aren't serving your body.

Don't feel guilty about throwing out "food" that's poisoning your body because that's exactly what you're doing when you eat processed food. The more you realize that most of the foods sold today are not good for us, the easier it will be to train your mind and body to avoid them.

Fat Doesn't Make You Fat

Fat is an essential part of our diets and is critical for well being. Eating the right kind of fat at the right time will not make you fat, it will help you lose weight. Remember, it's insulin that drives energy to be stored into fat. Pure fat produces a negligible amount of insulin and doesn't turn on fat-storing mode.

Of the 3 macronutrients, fat contains more than double the amount of calories (energy) per gram compared to proteins and carbs. This makes fat much more satiating compared to carbs and proteins and tends to fill you up faster because it's so rich.

Don't be fooled though. It's not the calories that count. The hormonal implications of insulin and glucagon matter more. It is much harder to overeat fats like coconut oil in one meal compared to carbs like pasta. Fat is also essential for many hormones in the body, including testosterone and growth hormones, which help you burn fat, build muscle and stay young.

Saturated fats, like those found in grass-fed butter and coconut oil, are highly beneficial as every cell wall in your body is made up of saturated fats. It's important to separate carbs and fats when possible. Having a diet high in carbs and fats can cause a lot of inflammation along with weight gain.

Fat on its own isn't bad. When you eat an excess amount of carbs with fat, problems like heart disease can occur. Avoid hydrogenated vegetable oils like canola. Focus on getting cold-pressed olive, avocado and coconut oil. It's important to understand that fat is also a buffer for toxins. When you eat foods filled with substances that your body doesn't know how to handle, it shuttles them into fat cells, so they don't interfere with the rest of the body.

Rapid weight loss can lead to self-intoxication due to the release of toxins from the fat cells. When you lose weight quickly, you want to eat healthy food so your liver can have the nutrients on board to run detox pathways efficiently.

If you want to dig deeper into this, check out the book "Good Calories, Bad Calories" by Gary Taubes. He lays out the history and corruption behind why many people believe saturated fat is bad for you. I will say, there are experts on both sides of the saturated fat debate. See what serves your body best.

Recalibration

There is a destination/recalibration period that occurs when you detox yourself from processed foods and especially from carbs. As children of modern Western society, it's normal and acceptable to eat highly processed and sugary foods from a young age.

Growing up, I used to have macaroni for breakfast and would pour Aunt Jemima syrup all over them along with spreading pure sugar on top. When you're competing against years of habitually over-saturating your body with processed foods, it will take some effort in the beginning to overcome that inertia.

Your taste buds have likely been oversaturated with rich foods your whole life so much so that when you go to eat something like plain oatmeal or a carrot that has much less sugar, your mouth rejects it. Once you start going down the path of health and removing fake processed foods from your diet, you will genuinely start to enjoy real food. Foods you used to love and crave will no longer taste the same as the ones you pictured in your mind and your desire to eat them will go away.

Carb Heavy Foods

Here's a list of foods that you should be avoiding. This is not inclusive of everything. If you're not sure about a food, google its nutritional content to see if carbs are the dominant macronutrient in them.

- Pasta
- Rice
- Potatoes
- Sweet potatoes
- Yams
- Melons
- Mangos
- Apples
- Bananas
- Candy bars
- Ice Cream
- Oatmeal
- Quinoa
- Beans
- Pancakes
- Chips
- Pizza
- Hot Dogs (buns)
- Burgers (buns)
- Most stores bought sauces (ketchup, BBQ, Ranch)
- Dates
- Figs
- Dried Fruits
- Nuts

Refined carbs
Sugar
White Bread
White Rice
corn / syrup
Dextrose
fructose
wheat flour
Pizza Dough
syrup
cause a spike
in insulin.

Healing Emotional Eating

"If more information was the answer, we'd all be billionaires with perfect abs."

- Derek Sivers

If it were as simple as understanding everything in this book, everyone would be slim and trim. You and I both know it's not as simple as having more information. There is a dark side to weight gain that simply isn't addressed enough in our externally focused Western society. We need to look beyond the physical and the material by turning inwards.

For many people, including myself, eating has a massive emotional component that often leads to food addictions. Admitting we have habits and patterns that no longer serve us is the first step. Committing to ourselves to dive deeper into these in order to make a change is the next step.

It's my goal to provide you with as much information as is necessary to guide you, but you are the one that must walk through the door and do the inner work. Food addiction can be scary. During childhood, it's easy to develop patterns that use food as a security blanket and to eat our emotions away. It becomes a reflex to reach for ice cream when we feel low, much like a child reaches for their blanket to cover up and feel safe.

We all have patterns that do not serve us, whether we are aware of them or not. As a child, eating ice cream may have been a way to escape feeling negative emotions. This does solve the problem temporarily and makes you feel better, but it doesn't lead to a solution and only delays you having to deal with the underlying emotion.

I won't lie to you, fasting and cutting out carbs may be the hardest thing you've done in a while because you're removing the emotional safety blanket that food brings. Without this shield, you will be left to face the emotions and to start overcoming them in order to succeed.

For some people, food may be the only thing they feel they have control over. For others, it's a distraction from what's really going on in their life. Getting to the root of your addiction will help you overcome it. By shining a light on your shadows, you take away their power over you. If you ignore the darkness it will continue to grow.

The physical dimension is not what matters most when one is trying to lose weight. The underlying mental, emotional, and spiritual aspects that lead to why you do what you do in the physical world needs to be peeled back like an onion. Western society tends to ignore the mental, emotional, and spiritual aspects of a person. These aspects cannot necessarily be seen, but greatly impact the physical. To change the physical condition, it would be wise to address the other 75% of your being.

If you're ready to make a serious change and become the best version of yourself, you will have to go through whatever you're not addressing within your inner world. Fasting and cutting carbs will take you to that edge. It's your choice whether you want to look over the cliff, jump and face your fears or remain in the same position you are in now.

Figuring out the function that food is playing in your life is an important step. Bringing mindfulness to your eating habits and presence with your meals is part of the process. The role food plays is different for everyone. You may or may not know yet what you are trying to avoid when you eat out of instinct or craving. The final section of this book will show you several ways to tune into your body and listen for answers.

How to Start

I wish I could magically tell you what problem you have right now and give you the solution for it but there are so many possibilities that I'd be here all day writing my guesses. Regardless of the problem, you have the solution inside you. Here is an exercise you can do that will start this process.

When you feel an emotion, craving, or uneasy feeling, focus on it. Locate the sensation in your body. Is it a tightness in your chest? Pressure in your head? Knots in your stomach? Perhaps a nagging chronic pain in your lower back? Once you locate it, focus on it. You can ask questions or you can just observe it with kindness and curiosity.

Do not get angry or upset with these sensations. Allow what's there to be fully expressed. Avoid repressing or judging any feelings and emotions. Remember that pain is a teacher. It's there to guide you. That uneasy feeling you're experiencing might be the pain teacher telling you to quit your job, get out of a relationship, or change whatever life circumstance that's not serving you.

We've all been in a situation that we knew wasn't good for us. Perhaps it's staying with a partner for too long due to fear of the unknown. We know that the relationship isn't nurturing our soul yet we stay there for security. We feel it like a bowling ball sitting in the pit of our stomachs. You might even experience it as a heaviness in your heart.

Maybe it's a job you hate that sucks the life and will to live out of you. Perhaps you get headaches constantly or have to take antacids because the stress is causing you heartburn. Stop putting that inner voice in silence and let it help guide you in life.

This method of listening to the body is what I personally used to overcome irritable bowel syndrome. My stomach used to go into severe pain even if I hadn't eaten something. It pissed me off constantly and made me angry. It wasn't until I was able to be present with the pain that I realized it was signaling my mental, emotional, and spiritual state. It showed me how the other 75% of my being was manifesting in my physical body.

I'm grateful for my IBS because, although it brought me pain for several years, it taught me a valuable lesson in listening to my body. My stomach is on the radar for trouble in life and has helped guide decisions with regards to relationships and work. I know that if it starts acting up around certain people or topics, there is a reason for it. You will have your own pains to listen to. The sooner you choose to acknowledge what's there, the faster you will grow and become who you truly want to be.

Bridge the Gap

1) Make your first meal of the day protein based. If you're a vegetarian or vegan, you should still focus your first meal on some sort of plant-based protein. Avoid carbs as your first meal.

2) Use Stevia if you absolutely need some sweetness in your drinks. Be aware it may trigger insulin because your brain is tasting the sweetness and in anticipation it can release insulin. Don't become reliant on it, use it as a tool to wean yourself off of sugar.

3) Add cinnamon to foods. Along with adding some sweetness to your meal, it can help stabilize and regulate blood sugar levels.

4) Switch out sweats/candy for 90% dark chocolate. It's an acquired taste, but trust me, you can acquire it. I used to absolutely hate the taste of it, but I used this same strategy and have now come to enjoy dark chocolate. You can start with 70% and work your way up. The darker the chocolate, the less sugar it tends to have.

5) Replace candy bars, chips, ice cream (simple/processed sugars) with fruits (complex and less processed sugars). Instead of reaching for a chocolate bar, have apples, bananas, strawberries, blueberries, or watermelons instead

6) Stop drinking anything with calories (other than bone broth). Liquids trigger the fastest and biggest response to insulin. Bone broth (vegan or regular) can help satisfy cravings for salty foods. It's also great for your digestion, skin, and overall health.

#4 PROTEIN POWER

"For a slim, sexy body, it's important to eat protein every day - preferably at every meal. Be sure to ask about the origins of your meat, poultry and seafood. If you can't afford organic, free-range meats, opt for natural poultry, pork, and beef that's raised without antibiotics or hormones."

- Suzanne Somers

In 2021, I decided to experiment with an almost exclusively carnivore diet. I cut out 95% of my carb intake for 6 weeks and focused on eating protein as the basis of every meal. The only exceptions were eating a few carrots and celery stalks here and there along with bone broth. This led to one of the craziest physical, mental, emotional, and spiritual transformations I'd experienced in such a short window of time.

During this diet, my energy levels skyrocketed. I became unstoppable. I had so much energy that it became difficult for me to go to sleep even after a really busy day. My sleep quality went down the toilet during this time as it took me forever to fall asleep and I would wake up around 5am automatically. The weird thing was that I wasn't tired.

After weeks of bad sleep, I would wake up every morning feeling refreshed and ready to take on the day. The energy dips that caused me to take a nap after eating a meal of rice or sweet potatoes were gone. On top of that, I became super lean. I was eating massive quantities of meat and the weight was flying off me. Without carbs, my body became a fat-burning machine. I'm not suggesting you need to go to this extreme, but it was interesting to see the effects of it on my body.

The Best Protein

If you want to maximize your ability to adhere to and take advantage of the previous 3 sections, meat, and particularly organ meat is one of the best ways I know how. It's jam packed with vitamins, minerals, and all sorts of nutrients that will satiate and fulfill your body's needs with a relatively small serving. Meat is much more satiating compared to carbs and doesn't increase insulin as much as carbs. This is especially true for organ meats.

If you're a vegetarian/vegan and don't want to eat animals, I fully respect your choice to not eat animals and maybe this section isn't for you. I'm not here to convince you to change or bash your ideologies. I simply ask that you read this section with an open heart and mind.

The goal of this entire book is to invite everyone, vegan, vegetarian, carnivore, paleo, keto, whatever diet you're currently following or not following to look in the mirror and be honest with yourself.

Is what you're eating serving you or is it hurting you?

Do you truly feel alive, vibrant, and happy eating what you're eating? Or are you committed to your diet because you have ideas and beliefs about it or the people telling you to do it? Maybe you're running on autopilot, eating what you've always eaten.

Some of you may have a problem eating animals because traditional factory farming causes animals to suffer and harms the environment. I don't support this either. You might consider learning to hunt or find farmers you trust that raise animals with their welfare in mind.

If your purpose in life is to help animals, restore the environment, or help the planet in some way, you need to be healthy and energetic in order to fight off the evils of this world that seek to do the opposite. If there is something missing in your diet that hinders your health, why not try introducing it to see what happens.

Eating a little bit of organ meat from an animal that was hunted could help you have vibrant energy and health, thus allowing you to better serve your purpose. That's why I'm focusing on organ meats in this section. You don't need to eat a lot of it to get the benefits. This reduces your impact plus saves you money.

I invite you to remove the dogmas and "isms". Evaluate each individual food on its own merit and listen to your body when you eat it to see if it's beneficial. Don't dogmatically apply rigid principles in what you eat because a book (like mine), expert, or friend told you it was good or forbid you from eating it.

Organ meat is a fantastic way to do that as you can really notice the nutrition it gives you through the satiation you receive after eating it. You don't need to eat a large quantity of organ meat to feel full, unlike eating a large steak or a rack of ribs smothered in BBQ sauce. Small quantities of organ meat go a long way.

Contrasted against other foods like popcorn, chips, or ice cream (all heavy in carbs), organ meat is extremely difficult to over consume and mindlessly eat. Organ meat is also very affordable since you don't need to buy as much and even the organic version sells for less than the cost of factory meat.

I suggest going to an organic butcher, farmer's market, or asking some hunters you may know in order to get your meat. You always want to get quality meat from an animal that was either raised ethically and allowed to graze on its natural food or an animal from the wild.

Animals raised in Concentrated Animal Feeding Operations (CAFOs) do not provide good quality meat. They are often stuck in small fenced areas, walking on their feces, and living unhappy lives. They are fed unnatural diets and injected with antibiotics constantly because they live in such dirty conditions.

Organic grass-fed meat has several benefits over their CAFO raised brethren. Grass-fed animals are allowed to roam outdoors and eat their natural diets which helps keep them happy and healthy. It's also better for the environment as the animals help to regenerate the soil and grasslands which in turn helps remove carbon from the atmosphere and return it to the soil.

Alongside that, grass-fed meat has higher nutritional value. For example, grass-fed beef has much higher levels of omega-3 fatty acids which help reduce inflammation and less omega-6 fatty acids. A high ratio of omega-6 to omega-3 is what leads to inflammatory damage from these fatty acids. Grass-fed beef is also an excellent source of conjugated linoleic acid which has powerful antioxidant effects.

Grass-fed beef is also superior in delivering more vitamins and minerals compared to conventional CAFO beef. It has more magnesium, calcium, potassium, zinc, beta-carotene, phosphorus, and iron compared to grain-fed beef. It also has more vitamin A, D, E, and K as well as higher levels of B vitamins.

Organic organ meat is especially potent. Alongside elevated levels of vitamins and minerals, organ meat such as beef heart is rich in an enzyme called CoQ10 which supports heart health, mitochondria, and blood pressure. The heart contains 4 times the amount of CoQ10 compared to muscle meat. It also has twice the elastin and collagen which aids in connective tissue and joint health.

Eating spleen is another excellent choice. It supports your immune health through its ability to build blood as it is a concentrated source of heme iron. Peptides such as splenopentin and tuftsin help to stimulate macrophages (defense cells) and neutrophils (a type of white blood cell). A deficiency in tuftsin may also be linked to bacterial infections.

The liver is a major source of nutrition and is nature's multi-vitamin. It's packed with folate, B-vitamins, iron, magnesium, zinc, selenium, potassium, and vitamins A, D, E, and K to name a few. This helps to support your immune system, metabolism, and detox pathways.

Some of you may have heard that you can overload yourself with vitamin A by eating too much liver. In the absence of adequate vitamin D, if you were to consume 300,000 IU (international units), you could get vitamin A toxicity. 1oz of grass-fed beef liver contains 5,000 IUs of vitamin A. That means you would have to eat 60oz (3.75lbs) of liver to achieve this.

As with anything in life, the dose makes the poison. I doubt anyone here was going to jump into eating nearly 4lbs of liver on day one, but I have to make sure. These really are like multivitamins. You don't need a large quantity to get a big effect. A few ounces a day with your meals is plenty.

The effects of food go beyond just the measurable micronutrient content. If you eat an animal that was sick, dying, and unhappy, you are absorbing that animal's negative energy. Eating something that has a low vibration will not aid in raising your levels of vitality. Whenever possible, do your best to buy meat that was raised well or hunted.

Going Inward

"Easy choices, difficult life. Hard choices, easy life. "

- Jerzy Gregorek

The easy path has you doing the same thing, day after day. This rewarding path has you going inward to see what is truly needed. There are many things that factor into your ability to eat certain foods and they can change from day to day.

Many factors will impact your ability to digest and more importantly absorb food. If you worked out, slept poorly, are under stress, haven't eaten in days etc. will play a role in digestion. Some people do well on a high vegetable and fruit diet while others do much better on a meat based diet.

The ability for your body to utilize the food you take in differs greatly depending on your entron length. The entron runs from mouth to anus and varies from person to person. If you have a longer entron, your ability to digest fibrous veggies will increase.

Just as cows have multiple stomachs in order to digest grass, humans with longer intestines have more time to digest and absorb the nutrients from plants compared to those with a short entron. Likewise, if someone with a long entron was to focus on a carnivore style diet, the meat may stay too long inside their intestines leading to excess fermentation.

If you've ever had protein shakes and noticed your farts smell worse after, this is a similar phenomenon. The protein in the shake didn't digest well and was fermenting in your digestive system, causing you gas and possibly bloating. The longer it takes to come out, the longer it can cause problems.

There are far too many differences between people to be able to suggest that one diet is optimal for everyone. That's why learning to tune into your body is so crucial.

Tuning Into Your Body

Here are some ways for you to see what foods are good for you. Experiment with your meals and treat them with a curious and explorative attitude. Keep in mind that just because you determine food is good for you today, doesn't mean it can't and won't change tomorrow. Your body is dynamic and constantly evolving. A diet or food that worked in the past, may not work the same today.

It's all practice. There is no "doing it wrong". As long as you're engaging with the practice, you are learning and taking an important step forward in your health. Here are some techniques to tune into your body and find out what works for you.

1. During and after your meal, tune into your body. If you're experiencing negative symptoms, you know something in your food isn't serving you.

2. Mindful eating. Not only will this help you find what foods are good for you, it will also help improve digestion.

   - Eat as slow as you can

- Chew as much as possible

- Engage with your taste buds

- Put utensil down between bites

- Avoid screens/distractions while eating

- Avoid stressful environments (eating at your desk/workspace)

- Say a prayer, blessing, or thanks to your food.

3. Limit the amount of ingredients in a meal. The more ingredients there are, the harder it will be to determine which ones are causing you a problem.

4. Eat one food at a time and tune into the sensations from that food. By spending a few minutes eating just one food, you can see the effects of it much better.

5. Figure out the specific needs behind any emotional eating. Is there an underlying emotion that comes up when you get a craving for a certain food? Can you locate where you feel it in your body? If you can, focus on it and see what comes through.

6. Inspect your stool. That's right, look into the toilet after you go to the bathroom. If your stool doesn't look like a decent sized sausage, light brown, with minimal smell, something is off. There's a reason many animals smell their bowel movements. They're checking to see what's up with their body. Undigested food particles, diarrhea, mucus, blood, constipation, and foul   smells are all signs that something you've eaten isn't mixing well with your body.

7. Use a diet log. One of the easiest ways to keep track of how a food affects you is to write it down. I've provided an example on the next page. You can use a journal and re-create it, or you can go here: Radoslav.ca/DietLog and download the pdf for free.

Food Diary

Date _____

M / Tu / W / Th / F / Sa / Su

Bedtime last night: Wake up time today: Hours slept:	Energy level upon waking: 1 2 3 4 5 6 7 8 9 10
Meal 1 Time _____ Observations:	Water • 500 ml • 1000 ml • 1500 ml • 2000 ml • 2500 ml • 3000 ml
Meal 2 Time _____ Observations:	Mood Morning:1 2 3 4 5 Afternoon:1 2 3 4 5 Evening:1 2 3 4 5
Meal 3 Time _____ Observations:	Exercise: Duration: • 15 mins • 30 mins • 45 mins • 60 mins
Snacks: Observations:	Things I'm Grateful for:
Notes:	One thing to improve:

Fungus and Parasites

In addition to the foods I have listed in the carb section, I highly suggest reading a simple 6 page PDF from my friend Michael Holt. He has put out a fantastic and concise resource on something known as an antifungal and antiparasitic diet. This PDF is the reason I decided to do 6 weeks of a carnivore focused diet. There are a lot of vegetable options available in the diet and it is by no means a meat exclusive diet. That's just how I did it.

If you experience cravings that you cannot solve, they can be coming from parasites and fungus. These invaders can release chemicals that stimulate cravings that would otherwise not be there. As long as you allow these unwelcome guests to stay, cravings and other health problems may persist.

Most people are unknowingly harboring a parasite, fungus, or both which is hindering their health. He does an excellent job describing exactly what to eat and why you should eat it. Alongside being an excellent diet to eliminate these parasites, his diet works incredibly well for losing weight as well due to its focus on eliminating almost all sugars and focusing on real food.

You can get his free 6-week protocol when you sign up to his email list at Radoslav.ca/FungusAndParasite. His recommendations are in line with what I've written here and if you follow his diet, you will see a huge shift in your health along with fat-loss.

Bridge the Gap

1. Supplements. The easiest way to take organ meat is to use pure organ meat supplements. I personally like the brand Higher Healths from Alberta, Canada. This is the most expensive option but if you have the means, it really simplifies the process of eating organ meats.

2. Slowly cook your organ meat. This will make it soft, tender, and easy to chew. The problem with many organ meats is that they tend to become chewy after you cook them. Put your organs into a slow cooker and leave them on low heat overnight.

3. Test out different organ meats from different animals. There are some organs you'll find you prefer more compared to others and they will taste different coming from another animal. Start with a spread of different organs/animals and see which ones suit you best. You do want to eat a wide variety of organ meats, but in the beginning, find your favorites and slowly keep adding.

4. Soak your organ meat in milk for 30-60 minutes. This will help remove the taste we've all come to associate with organ meats. Use salt, pepper, and any other seasoning you enjoy to help add flavor and make it easier to add to your diet.

5. Add a little bit of organ meat to your meals. You don't need to eat the entire organ in one sitting to get the benefits. Notice how even a few bites of organ meat impact your hunger and satiety.

6. Have organ meat with your first meal of the day and start by eating it first. You'll likely find that it's harder to overeat during meals where you begin with organ meat.

#5 LOSE WEIGHT WHILE YOU SLEEP

"Sleep is the best medication"

- Dalai Lama

Staying up until 1am and waking up at 7am was how I lived my life from childhood into my early 20s. I would be up late playing video games until my eyes couldn't stay open anymore. I was a screen addict. When I didn't need to wake up early, I would often stay up even later and wake up much later.

Alongside this came horrible eating patterns. Pizza, cereal, donuts, burgers, and candy were a major part of my diet. Bad food choices tend to go with staying up late. Perhaps you're someone who enjoys a midnight snack. Being up late will continue to encourage this behavior, ruin your fasting schedule, and keep you from achieving your body transformation goals.

This habit of staying up late and eating garbage food kept me in a low state of health. I was often sick, fatigued, and had a nose that was so stuffed up that I could barely breathe through it. I simply wasn't sleeping enough to allow my body to function properly. I don't really have to tell you that without good sleep your body just doesn't function well. You know it and can feel it.

The Best Medicine

Sleep is the best medicine for any remedy. This sacred time is where the body goes into a hyper drive to heal, repair, and recharge. Without sleep, many of your body's systems start working below their capability, making you feel slow, tired, and keeping you from losing weight.

Imagine only charging your phone to 33% battery capacity every night. You would spend all day trying your best to conserve energy and would never get full function from your phone. When you go to sleep, do you give your body the best chance to reach 100% charge? Or are you sabotaging yourself and living off of just a fraction of your potential?

Missing sleep and feeling tired makes it difficult to focus and do the things you need to do in order to lose weight. Sleep has a profound effect on your hormone cycle as well and can limit the amount of weight you lose. Not getting enough sleep is an added stressor to your body. In ancestral times, not being able to sleep often meant you were not in a safe environment. Your body was on high alert in order to keep you alive.

It's not as simple as just telling you to go to bed earlier and get more sleep. You likely know that already. What this section will take you through is a fundamental understanding of the advantages of better sleep and what you can do to improve your sleep quality and quantity that is beyond just going to bed at a certain time.

Your Rhythm is Off

Your body has a 24 hour hormonal cycle known as a circadian rhythm. This cycle is based on your sleep and wake times and is modulated by the signals you receive from the environment; ideally, from the sun and the moon. It helps your body know when to produce more energy and when to calm down.

In the morning, the sun rises and should hit your skin and eyes. This sends signals to your brain and body to wake up and become active through the release of cortisol. When the sun sets, our bodies are supposed to wind down, get ready for bed and for sleep. When we let this happen, melatonin is released to help us fall asleep.

If this cycle is running optimally, your body can harmonize all of its hormones allowing you to achieve a healthy state. Since we live in a modern society, we have jobs, technology, family, games, and screens of all kinds that manipulate our natural sleep-wake cycle, keeping us from getting adequate and deep sleep.

Quality and Quantity

Everyone is different in how much sleep they need. I tend to err on the side of suggesting that adding more sleep for most people will usually improve their health. However, this is not always true so judge for yourself where you fall within my recommendations.

7-9 hours is a rough estimate as to how many hours you need. In general, the younger you are, the more sleep you need. As you get older, you will tend to sleep less. 8 hours is a good amount of sleep to aim for in the beginning. If you notice your energy, mood, and weight improving then you know you've found a good amount of sleep.

If you're sleeping past 9 hours and constantly feel groggy and unable to get yourself out of bed, you may need to limit the amount of sleep you're getting or adjust your bedtime. Ideally, you would be going to bed around 10pm and waking up around 6am. From 10pm-2am, due to your body's circadian rhythm, your body is releasing a lot of hormones that will promote repairs to your physical body.

Hormones like testosterone and growth hormones are more potent during this time. If you're sleeping during this period, you're maximizing their ability to repair your muscles and burn your fat. If you're awake and skipping this crucial time, you're not allowing two of the most powerful hormones to keep you young and healthy.

From 2am-6am, your circadian rhythm will trigger hormones that work on repairing & recharging your brain for mental activities. If your goal is to have a healthy body, you need to do your best to be in bed and sleeping around 10pm so you don't miss this critical 4 hour window.

Since we have seasons, this will change a bit throughout the year and you should be flexible. In the summer, you may go to bed later as the sun is up much later and wake up earlier because it rises earlier. During the winter, you can go to bed earlier since it's darker outside for a longer period and wake up later.

Much like I suggested with food (and everything in this book), you will need to find your sweet spot and know that it will likely change throughout the year.

Less Sleep = More Weight Gain

Lack of sleep makes fat loss much harder as it puts your body into stress mode, raises cortisol and decreases your insulin sensitivity. Cravings become more intense and harder to control. Even if you eat less and fast, your hormone balance will likely be off, making it harder to lose weight.

There are two key hormones we have yet to talk about when it comes to losing weight. These hormones control your hunger and satiety sensations and are therefore crucial for your ability to adhere to any sort of diet or fasting schedule.

The first hormone is called leptin. Leptin is produced by your fat cells and helps give you the feeling of satiety or fullness. When your body is functioning well, this hormone reduces your appetite signal making it easier to go longer periods without feeling the need to eat.

Since this hormone is produced by fat cells, one might think that having more fat should cause your appetite to decrease as you have more cells producing the hormone. In healthy individuals, this may be the case. However, we can think of this as a state similar to those with diabetes.

In type 2 diabetes, which is about 90% of all diabetes, fat cells become desensitized to the effects of insulin. More and more insulin needs to be produced and in the case of diabetes not enough insulin can be produced which is why exogenous insulin needs to be injected into a person with the disease.

Similarly, if your body has become desensitized to leptin's appetite suppressing signal through excess eating, it can be hard for you to detect the signals being sent to you that are telling you

you're full. Emotional eating can be a cause of this as well and is therefore important to address using the tools in this book.

The hormone ghrelin works in the opposite direction as leptin. Ghrelin is produced by the stomach and sends your brain the signal that you're hungry. Alongside stimulating hunger and an increase in food intake, ghrelin can reduce your metabolism and promote the retention of fat.

When you have poor quality sleep or a general lack of sleep, your body reduces its output of leptin and increases the amount of ghrelin you produce. Thus making it harder to lose weight and to stave off cravings. That's right, less sleep means increased cravings and a reduction in your metabolism.

For a lifestyle change like fasting and reducing the intake of high carbohydrate processed foods to stick, take advantage of your hormones and don't let them take advantage of you. Improving sleep quality/quantity has as great of an impact on your health and weight as diet and exercise.

Insulin and Sleep

Poor sleep also leads to a reduction in insulin sensitivity. This means that you need more insulin to be produced in order to store the energy from your food. For example, if someone who's never drank alcohol before has 1-2 beers, they will be much more sensitive to them compared to someone who's been drinking for years and needs to drink more beer to feel it.

Likewise, someone who has been eating high sugar, carbs, and processed foods will need more insulin to continue forcing energy storage into fat cells. Insulin sensitivity plays an important role in weight loss and overall health. The higher your sensitivity, the less insulin you need to get the job done.

Less insulin means you can start using fat for energy sooner. More insulin equals more time spent in fat storing mode. This also increases cravings as insulin lowers blood sugar, which tricks your brain into thinking it needs to eat again.

Melatonin, Sleep, and Weight Loss

Melatonin is a critical hormone when it comes to sleeping. It's produced by your brain when you are in darkness. It helps to maintain your 24 hour circadian rhythm when it's allowed to function properly.

In the absence of (blue) light, you can create more melatonin and achieve a deeper and more restful sleep. Melatonin, however, isn't what causes you to sleep. It helps induce a state of quiet and peace that allows you to drift off into sleep.

It's important to understand that for every hour you spend in front of a screen (blue light) before bed, you're suppressing your melatonin release by about 30 minutes. That's right, if you spend 2 hours watching TV or scrolling instagram before bed, it can take an hour for melatonin to kick in after you stop remove the screen.

Melatonin is critical hormone that you will learn how to optimize and balance. Without it, deep and restful sleep can be difficult to achieve and as you've just read, bad sleep will throw off other hormones such as leptin, ghrelin, insulin, and cortisol.

On top of that, melatonin has the ability to help mobilize and activate something known as brown adipose tissue (BAT). Adipose is a fancy word for fat. BAT has a unique characteristic in that, unlike white adipose tissue, it has a much higher concentration of mitochondria. Mitochondria is considered the powerhouse of every cell where energy is generated. Regular white adipose tissue doesn't have nearly as much mitochondria as brown adipose tissue.

The more BAT you have and the more you can stimulate it, the more you raise your body's metabolism through its energy producing capacity. That's right, the more BAT you have, the more regular fat tissue you can burn for energy. The practicality of this type of tissue along with how to build it will be further discussed in the final section.

Sleeping Postures and Pillow Placements

The position in which you sleep will play a crucial role in your overall health. I can't count the amount of times I've had clients come in and tell me their shoulder or neck hurts and they don't know why. Upon further questioning, they would usually tell me that they slept with their arm extended in a weird position or their head was awkwardly twisted.

If you're staying in any position for a prolonged period of time, that position can have dire consequences. The position may be impinging or putting undue pressure onto a joint, especially if you are unconscious during that time and can't sense that you should move. While sleeping, you can achieve a position you would never think of holding while awake yet could be spending hours every night maintaining it.

Let's start with the worst position to sleep in and work our way up to the most ideal. You should do your best to avoid sleeping on your stomach as this puts your neck in a compromised position all night. Having your head fully turned to the left or right for long periods of time is a recipe for disaster when it comes to neck health. Maintaining a neutral neck will help prevent impingements along with pinched nerves. Sleeping on your stomach also tends to aggravate many peoples' lower back as it causes an excessive curvature in the lumbar region.

Sleeping on your side would be a step up from sleeping on your stomach. It is usually not ideal as you need several pillows placed properly in order to support your spine and hold it in a neutral position as shown in the picture. Neck, hip, and lower back pain can occur without proper pillow support for the head and knees. Even though this position is an improvement, the shoulder on which you are leaning on does take excess pressure and with time can aggravate the shoulder capsule causing pain.

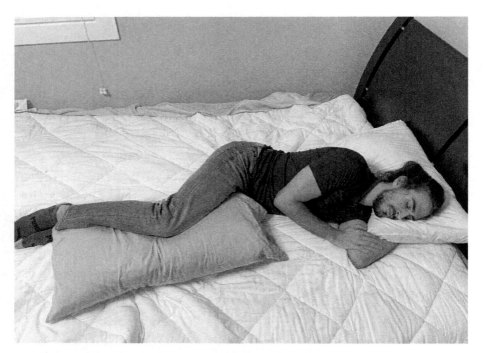

The ideal position to sleep in is on your back. This allows for a neutral spine and an even distribution of pressure throughout your body without any hotspots taking excessive tension. Maintaining good posture while sleeping is critical for joint and muscle health. There are two important pillows that will likely need to be modified here in order to achieve optimal alignment for your spine. The first is the most obvious, that being the one under your head.

You want to use the most minimal pillow or possibly no pillow to achieve a neutral curvature in your neck. If you have an excessive forward head posture, you will need a pillow to not strain your neck. If you have a tall and erect spine with an upright head posture, putting a pillow behind your neck may put you into an excessive forward head posture.

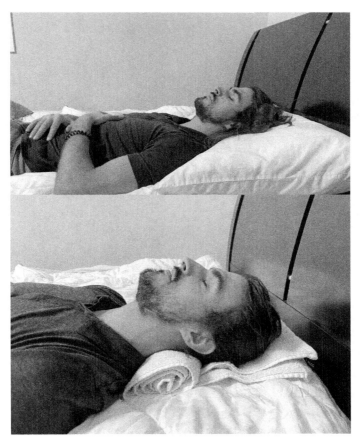

I've personally worked on my posture and sleeping position so that I do not require a pillow behind my head. It feels really awkward having one there now. You can gradually downgrade your pillow to a smaller and smaller one or you can use a rolled up towel to provide a little bit of support for your neck as you make these changes and adaptations.

The second pillow you will likely need to use will go under your knees. You'll need to experiment with its size to see what serves you best. Bending the knee helps unlock and take pressure off of your lower back. This helps prevent compression and tension from building up while you're sleeping.

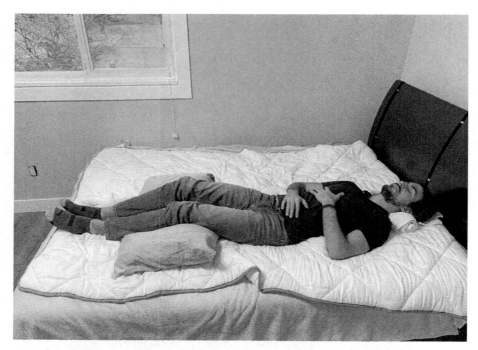

The more comfortable you can make your body, the easier it will be to sleep. Using these tips will also help reduce joint pressure and pain in your muscles. Sleep should recover and restore you, not cause you to wake up feeling sore and stiff. Most likely, you're going to struggle with sleeping on your back. It took me about 6 months of effort to feel comfortable sleeping on my back. If you have difficulty transitioning to this position, here's what I did to achieve it.

Commit the first 15-30 minutes of your sleep to being on your back. After that, switch to whatever position is most comfortable. As the weeks go by, you can extend that time to 1, 2, 3, etc. hours of the night. Gradually build yourself up to sleep in an optimal position. There is no sense in laying there for 4 hours like a mummy if you can't fall asleep.

Bridge the Gap

This section is going to be a little different. In order to maximize your hormonal advantages and get the most out of your sleep, I've provided a "best practices" list as well as some "sleep aids" to improve the quantity and quality of your sleep.

The best practices are 100% free. You can pick which ones you feel will be easy to add to your lifestyle. Sleep aids are things you can buy that will help enhance your ability to sleep at night.

Since there are so many variables to sleep, it's hard to say which one of these is the easiest or hardest to do since you are likely already doing some of these while excluding others. Pick the action items that you think will be the easiest for you to achieve and start putting them into practice.

Best Practices

1. Get up and get out of bed as soon as your alarm goes off. Do not hit the snooze button. When you hit the snooze button first thing in the morning, you're sending the signal to your brain that you don't want to get up and engage with life. When you have a clear purpose along with goals in life, waking up becomes much more exciting. Refer to the mindset and goal section to help you get excited to wake up.

2. Get out ASAP after getting out of bed. A few minutes of sun exposure in the morning can help set your circadian rhythm by stimulating cortisol, which also helps you wake up.

3. Don't have your cell phone next to you while you sleep. Leave your phone across the room. When your alarm goes off, it forces you to get up to turn it off.

4. Use airplane mode before bed. Don't allow people to reach you at 1am in the morning. The last thing you need is a "DING" to interrupt your sleep and trigger a stress response.

5. Avoid going to bed later on weekends. Your body thrives on having a routine. If you go to bed at 10pm Monday to Thursday, but 2am or 3am on Friday, Saturday, and Sunday it throws off your body's circadian rhythm. It induces an almost jet-lag type of chaos, shifting your body-clock several hours every weekend. By the time Thursday comes around and your body has finally adjusted from the weekend, it has to start the process all over again. Do your best to avoid this.

6. Commit to waking up at the same time every morning, regardless of what time you went to bed. This will help keep you honest with your bedtime and will help your body get into a routine. The earlier you wake up, the easier it is to go to bed at night.

7. Your mentality around sleep is very important. Some people, including myself, can get anxiety over sleep, especially if you have or have had problems sleeping in the past. Setting the intention to have a good sleep and wake up with energy can help. If you go to bed thinking that you won't sleep well and you will wake up tired, you are creating a self-fulfilling prophecy. Set the expectation that you will get up eagerly and with energy in order to achieve your goals.

8. Use the last 30-60 minutes of your day to connect with family or people in your household. If you sleep with a partner, you can massage each other's hands and feet before bed. This will help both of you relax and get closer with each other.

9. Stretch before bed. A few simple stretches before bed can help calm your nervous system and relax your body. I recommend taking a couple of minutes and stretching out any tight muscles, especially your chest and hip flexors.

10. Avoid doing anything other than sleep or having sex in your bedroom if possible. You don't want to condition your mind and body by doing work or anything mentally stimulating in bed.

11. Keep your room clean. A messy room can hold a lot of chaotic energy that stimulates your body. I find that burning sage in my room and house after cleaning helps to relax my body tremendously by clearing out dense energy from the environment.

12. If you workout in the morning, even just for 5-15 minutes, it can help align your cortisol levels and circadian rhythm. Should you wake up groggy in the morning and feel the need for a caffeine boost, engage in a morning power walk before coffee and see how your energy feels after.

13. Avoid napping, especially after 2pm. This can mess with your ability to fall asleep at night as well as with your circadian rhythm. If you must nap, limit it to 15 minutes by using an alarm. Do some deep breathing during this time to help re-energize your body.

14. Limit liquid intake a few hours before bed. You don't want a full bladder to wake you up throughout the night.

15. Avoid having caffeinated drinks like coffee after 1pm. Some people metabolize coffee quickly while others take a much longer time. If you drink coffee, do your best to limit its intake after 1pm to make sure the caffeine isn't keeping you awake

16. Having a ritual or routine you follow before going to bed can help condition your body to start relaxing once it recognizes that it's going to bed soon. You can write down a simple routine by picking out a few of the actions listed here. The more straightforward it is, the easier it will be to follow. You don't need to start

with a 1 hour routine. Even a 5 minute practice before bed will be beneficial.

17. Avoid news, Instagram, work emails or anything that may stress you out. You don't want any stimulation (good or bad) before bed and you especially don't want new information that you can't do anything about swirling around your mind while you try to sleep.

18. Reduce the temperature in your room. If it's too hot and you're uncomfortable, your body will not be able to relax. Play with the temperature and experiment to find out what is best for you. Perhaps cracking open the window or using a different set of sheets will make your body more comfortable and better able to sleep.

19. Take a hot or cold shower before bed. Depending on the season and climate of your home, taking a temperature focused shower can help enhance your sleep. If you're in a cold climate, taking a warm shower before bed may help you sleep. If you're in a warm climate, a cold shower can help you cool down and sleep better. Experiment to see which provides the best results for you.

20. Simple tools like earplugs and an eye mask can be the missing link to better nights sleep. If you live in a noisy area or can't control how much light is in your room, these are not only going to help you fall asleep but they will help you stay asleep.

Sleep Aids

1. If you have a hard time sleeping because you have too many thoughts in your head, keep a journal or notepad by your bed. Write down things you need to remember for the next day, schedules or anything that your brain deems important enough to keep replaying. If you can't sleep because something is bothering you emotionally, write that down. The act of writing it helps to release it from you and helps give you a better view of the situation at hand.

2. Set up blue light blocking software on your device. Blue light stimulates cortisol and stops the body from producing melatonin. Set night mode on your computer and cell phone. Software such as F.Lux and Twilight helps to reduce the blue light that comes from your device.

3. Use blue light blocking glasses at night and even at work if you stare at a computer all day. Don't buy the blue light reflecting glasses. Specialty yellow tinted glasses work well during the daytime with computer use. Orange tinted glasses are ideal for nighttime use to help protect your melatonin.

4. Use Himalayan salt lamps to light your home at night. Not only are they pretty, they also emit an orange tinted light which is akin to fire. The orange light will help to maintain your melatonin production vs regular ceiling lights and lamps that produce a harsh bright blue light.

5. Make your room as dark as possible. Don't have LED clocks or any light emitting devices in your room. If you have excessive light pollution coming into your room, consider buying black out curtains. The less artificial light that hits you, the better your melatonin production will be.

6. Try using herbal tea for sleep. Usually brand name teas will have a blend of the following ingredients which have sleep enhancing properties: lavender, valerian root, chamomile, magnolia, and passion flower. Experiment and see which one's work best with your body.

7. Using essential oil sprays can have similar effects to drinking tea. You can buy lavender essential oil spray. Be sure to buy from reputable dealers that don't use fillers or artificial substances.

8. If you feel hungry at night, you can drink bone broth to help satiate you or carbonated water. I've found that if I have a hot drink before bed, it causes me to become hot and sweat. When I drink cold carbonated water before bed, it helps cool me down and improves my sleep. Experiment with their temperatures for yourself to see what serves you best.

9. If you're like me, a heavy comforter or even a weighted blanket can be useful. The extra pressure can help to calm your body and ground you. You can also put a pillow on top of your torso if you sleep on your back.

#6 WALKING YOUR HUMAN

"I took a walk in the woods and came out taller than trees."

- Henry David Thoreau

It takes me a great deal of motivation and energy to get myself to go for my daily walks. After spending many years training my body to sit in one position as I played video games, overcoming the inertia of a sedentary lifestyle in order to leave my home didn't come naturally to me. However, by connecting the results of the walk to the benefits I receive I am able to overcome years of programming.

Walking is an indispensable tool for my mental and physical health. Going out provides a peace of mind that is matched by very few things. Walking in nature helps boost my creativity and is what got me through writing this book. I am not a writer by nature and much of this book was written after I went out for a walk.

I have never returned home from a walk feeling worse than when I left. Walking will be a tool you can access daily to reinvigorate yourself and to lose weight. There are a host of benefits and theories I can give you, but it is also something you will have to just try for yourself in order to understand. If you're not already taking daily walks, it's time to add this incredible habit to your routine.

I called this section "Walking Your Human" for a very specific reason. I think of the body as a dog and your mind is the owner. If you don't take your dog out for a walk, he or she won't be happy. He will bark, make a mess, and misbehave because there is no outlet for the pent-up energy.

Taking care of yourself is similar to taking care of a dog. You need to let them out in nature. They must be allowed to move their body. Treat yourself like a dog and walk your human daily.

Don't allow yourself to be trapped in a cage all day without letting yourself loose every once in a while.

The Power of a Walk

Never underestimate the power of walking in nature. We spend so much of our lives plugged into devices that we take very little time to connect with ourselves and nature. Having a daily practice of going out (especially in the morning) can help you tune into yourself, calm your nervous system, and turn on your Fat-Burning Mode.

Walking in the morning is ideal as your body has depleted its stores of liver glycogen overnight, making you better able to access your fat stores. Insulin has leveled off and glucagon has started to kick in to release energy from your fat cells.

As you walk in the morning, your heart rate goes up and the demand for energy to be produced is increased (your metabolism goes up). This demand for energy combined with your fasted state and glucagon in your blood stream makes it the ideal way to burn fat.

To better understand why walking is so important, I'm going to give you a brief, day 1 physiology lesson so you can truly know the benefits of walking for fat loss. You will also have an understanding of your body that 99% of people don't know.

Your Energy Systems

Your body has 3 systems it uses to produce energy. All three work together, it's never just one system acting alone. However, based on the demands you're putting onto your body, a different system will do the bulk of the work. Let's look at 3 examples from sports to help you understand what is going on in your body.

In the world of running, we have a wide range of distances one can compete in. You have likely engaged with these in some capacity, so you'll be able to understand what is going on. If we look at the 100m, 400m, and 26.1 mile (marathon) distances, we can use them to understand the 3 systems that are at work in our bodies.

The energy system that your body will use for its primary fuel source will depend on the amount of energy you demand from it. If you want to run faster, you are implying that you are moving towards 100% of your effort at any given moment. If you want to run slower, you are moving away from 100% effort.

Stated another way, you wouldn't take a leisurely pace while racing 100m and you wouldn't do an all-out sprint during the first 100m of a marathon race. The scenarios below are based on you trying to get the best time possible by taking advantage of each energy system.

Generally speaking, the more output you demand relative to 100% of your effort, the faster you will burn through your energy reserves and feel fatigued. Hence, you can walk (low demand) all day but sprint all out for short periods of time and for a limited amount of attempts.

At 100m, the primary energy system working is known as the anaerobic alactic system. It is also known as the ATP-CP system. Anaerobic means your body is producing energy without oxygen. Alactic means your body isn't using lactic acid either.

The 100m distance demands a massive amount of energy for a short period of time. In order to produce the amount of energy needed for this burst of energy, a molecule known as Adenosine Triphosphate (ATP) is broken down into Adenosine Diphosphate (ADP). This breakdown releases energy, allowing your muscle to receive fuel for the work it's doing.

Another molecule known as Creatine Phosphate (CP) is located in the muscle as well. When ATP breaks down into ADP, CP can separate itself in order to donate a phosphate to ADP. ADP and CP come together to recreate the starting molecule of ATP in order to continue giving energy.

This process takes place in the local muscle that needs energy. It is immediate energy that is accessed when a high demand is placed on the body. You want to run 100m in under 10 seconds? You need a lot of energy in a short period of time. Much like hitting a nitric oxide button in a car, you can burn up a lot of fuel in a short period of time to produce a lot of energy.

To recap, the anaerobic alactic or ATP-CP energy system is for short burst or high intensity efforts where a lot of energy is demanded over a short period of time. The energy is stored and accessed directly in the working muscle, and the fuel tank lasts for about 8-12s at 100% effort. The other 2 systems are contributing to the effort but their ability to generate enough energy in a short period is inferior to the ATP-CP system.

This is why you cannot keep sprinting at 10m/s for much longer than 100m. There is only a limited supply of ATP-CP in your muscles. Once this runs out, your body can't hit peak performance in output and starts to rely on an intermediate system.

Another example of this would be when you're lifting a heavy weight. You can only lift a heavy weight so many times before your muscle fatigues and you're unable to lift it. The energy has run out and you can no longer produce as much output as when your ATP-CP stores were at full. It takes about 3-5 minutes for you to refill your muscles. Your recovery will be based on your training and how much effort you put forth.

As we change the distance (aka the energy demand constraints), the dominant energy system changes. At 400m, the body starts relying on the anaerobic lactic system. This is also known as the glycolytic (sugar burning) system. Again we see the word anaerobic which means no oxygen is involved but this time we have lactic acid available.

This system tends to last anywhere from 30-120 seconds depending on how hard you are going, how much training you have, and how much pain you're willing to endure. We can simplify the lactic acid system by thinking of your energy as a bank account. The numbers I'm about to use are hypothetical and for explanation purposes only.

In order to run 400m in a certain time period, let's say 70 seconds, you will need to use 1,000 credits worth of energy. Let's say your energy system alone can produce 600 credits and you can borrow 400 credits that will be paid back at a later time. The extra 400 credits of debt come in the form of lactic acid. Several factors affect your glycolytic energy system. The more trained you are, the fresher you are, the more fed you are and the higher your pain tolerance is, the deeper you can go into debt by building up lactic acid.

You may have experienced this before when you gave 110% during an exercise or run. You likely ended up on the floor for several minutes gasping for air trying to recover. What's happening here? You've stopped demanding energy from your body as you're just laying down, but yet you're completely wiped for a period of time after.

This is what happens when you dig into the anaerobic lactic acid system. You go into energy debt by accumulating lactic acid. You know this is a painful process as you've no doubt felt this at least once in your life. Whether it's sprinting 400m or lifting a heavy weight for 8-12 reps.

The main fuel source for this system is sugar. That's right, those carbs you've been eating go directly into fueling these high intensity efforts. Sugar is vital for high intensity sports and for weightlifting. The lactic acid energy system is known as the glycolytic energy system because it uses the sugar stored in the muscle cells to generate energy.

That leaves us with the final energy provider known as the aerobic energy system. This system relies on converting oxygen and fat cells into energy. For most daily activities and leisures, this is the primary system providing you with energy. It can provide a large amount of energy over a long period of time as long as the effort is relatively low.

Fat, unlike the previous two systems, is burned from all over the body to provide energy, not the muscle or area of the body you are using. Many people make the mistake of thinking that if they do 1,000 crunches a day they will burn belly fat. This couldn't be farther from the truth and there are much better ways to burn belly fat.

While the ATP-CP and lactic acid systems use energy directly from the muscle, fat energy is consumed based on your genetics. The first place you tend to gain weight in (hips, thighs, stomach or face) is usually the last place you lose it from. This is why we have people with more apple, pear, or hourglass shapes.

There are very practical ways to manipulate exercise to maximize fat loss and not spin your wheels. We will be applying everything you've just learned so you understand the power of walking in nature, but later, I will touch on how this applies to working out as well.

If you were to do a long distance race such as a marathon, your fat and oxygen burning (aerobic) system would deliver a large amount of energy for that effort. From the previous example, if you're trying to run 400m in 70 seconds, you need 1,000 credits of energy. The energy needed for a marathon will be much different.

If you're running a marathon, then perhaps every 400m will take you 210 seconds to complete as you're trying to conserve energy for the entire race. In this case, the 400m may only cost you 150 credits of energy. You are trying to avoid using up all your sugar and ATP-CP stores so you don't go into energy debt, which would have you panting and feeling your muscles burning.

You may have heard of the marathoner who "hits the wall". This phenomenon usually takes place around the halfway mark or roughly 2 hours but can vary greatly depending on many factors. This happens because the lactic acid system has consumed a vast majority of its energy reserves and your body can no longer create enough energy to move at a pace that was previously sustainable.

Fat tissue can easily store 50,000 calories of energy in even a lean person. Depending on your muscle mass, training and food intake you can only hold onto about 500g carbs (2,000 calories) in your muscles and 100g (400 calories) in your liver, assuming you're fully fed.

Once those carbs run out, your ability to generate energy is severely reduced, making it feel incredibly hard to keep running if you haven't trained your body properly. When you train, whether it's weightlifting, running, tennis, or just plain old walking, you are training these energy systems based on the specific demand of the activity.

If you wanted to become a faster sprinter, you would train sprinting, not walking. The opposite is true. If you wanted to run a marathon, you wouldn't just train sprinting because they are opposite energy systems. Your body adapts to the loads and challenges you put on it. This is where you can take advantage of this new knowledge. Let's put it all together with a few more examples.

Why Traditional Weight Loss Classes Suck

Most likely, you have been to an exercise class that has focused on high intensity interval training (HIIT). There are many names for it, but the basics of it is that you're trying to get your heart rate up through vigorous movement. HIIT classes usually have you moving and sweating a lot with the intention of burning off as many calories in that class as possible.

I generally don't recommend people do these classes for a multitude of reasons. Primarily, people tend to get injured when doing things for the sole intention of raising their heart rate, especially if they haven't been taught proper form.

The other reason I don't recommend it is because of its

negligible weight loss impact. It can make many other things harder. Due to their intensity and high energy demand, they primarily use the ATP-CP and lactic acid energy system. The aerobic system is active during this, but it cannot provide the level of energy needed during one of these typical classes and your body relies heavily on the other two systems.

This type of high heart rate training consumes muscle mass if there isn't an emphasis on strength or muscle building exercises with adequate weights. You'll learn later why it's critical to keep as much muscle mass as you can while losing weight.

You just learned that high energy demanding exercise focuses on burning fuel (sugar) located in the muscles. Your goal is to burn calories from fat cells in order to reduce your weight. You don't want to deplete your muscle energy stores just for the sake of burning those calories. If you're not actively focusing on building strength or muscle, this type of training can be a waste of time.

When training, you want to maximize accessing fat stores, building strength, or creating new muscle. Elevating your heart rate for the sake of burning calories is a poor way to achieve long term fat loss results. If you want to lose weight, you need to work smarter, not just harder.

The other major downside to this style of training is that it puts your body into stress mode and increases food cravings. If you just burned off 500 calories and then go reward yourself with a high calorie meal, you've undone all your hard work.

You want to focus on training that makes you burn fat and while not increasing your cravings for high calorie food, which HIIT training tends to do. Realize that by training this way, you're ramping up your body's lactic acid energy system which relies on sugar. Your body wants to replace that sugar as quickly as possible in case you need to use your muscles again soon after.

Unless you're an athlete or training to build muscle, you don't need to be focusing on improving this energy pathway as your primary source of fuel. You want to train your body to burn fat and to be able to produce more energy from it so you can burn it off faster.

Your physiology lesson is now over. If you understand this basic model of the 3 energy systems in your body, you now know how to properly focus on fat-loss with any activity you do.

Burning the Most Amount of Fat Possible

Fasted low intensity cardio (walking/jogging) allows you to optimize for burning fat during and after exercise through the magic of enzymes. Enzymes are proteins that help speed up metabolism. Through walking or even a light jog, you can start to command your body to produce more fat burning enzymes.

If you increase the amount of fat burning enzymes your body has, you can produce more energy from the increased metabolization of fat when energy is demanded. Keep in mind, if you're engaging with traditional HIIT classes, jacking up your heart rate, and focusing on your glycolytic (sugar) burning system, you are asking your body to increase its sugar burning enzymes rather than fat burning enzymes.

Years ago, I came across a book by Mark Sisson called "Primal Endurance". After reading it, I decided to train my cardio and fat burning system using his recommendations. I highly recommend his book for anyone that wants to improve their cardio and their overall health.

Mark related one's heart rate to their energy system. As your heart rate rises, you are asking for more energy from your body and are therefore moving towards the lactic acid and the ATP-CP system. The lower your heart rate, the more you rely on fat as your primary fuel source.

His recommendation, baring injuries and other ailments, is to take your age and subtract it from 180 to find the lactic threshold at which you should peak in terms of heart rate.

The lactic threshold is where your body starts producing more lactic acid than it can remove, meaning that you are now accumulating lactic acid debt and will likely slow down soon or your heart rate will keep rising.

As you pass through your lactic threshold, you are focusing on consuming sugar as your primary fuel source and are not prioritizing your fat burning system anymore. The closer you can stay to your threshold without going over, the more you are stimulating your body to create fat burning enzymes.

Here's what that looked like for me. Keep in mind that you don't need to jog or even want to improve your ability to run. This example will show you how powerful the fat burning system can be if you train it properly through low intensity exercise.

Example for a 23 year old (my age when I read the book)

180 - 23 = 157 beats per minute (bpm)

If you want to be sure you're staying below your lactic threshold, using a heart rate monitor is the best idea. However, you don't absolutely need one. You can also gauge by your ability to talk or your ability to breathe through your nose. If you can talk while walking or jogging, you are below your lactic threshold. If you can breathe through just your nose, you are also likely to be below your lactic threshold as well.

During my experiments with this method, my first recorded 30 minute run while limiting my heart rate below 157bpm came out to a distance of 4.07km with an average heart rate of 152bpm. It's also a stretch to use the word "running" here. Most of it was done at a moderate walk as anytime I started running, my heart rate shot past 157bpm.

After 2 months of doing this training while keeping my heart rate down, I tested my 30 minute time again. During this effort, I covered 4.75km in 30 minutes while maintaining an average of 146bpm. I went further, without stopping to walk and with a lower heart rate.

I remember having to force myself to run harder in order to raise my heart rate. After just 2 months of training a few days a week at this low effort, my body's ability to produce energy while keeping my heart rate down had drastically improved.

Being able to run a further distance at the same time while simultaneously reducing my heart rate by 6 beats shows an improvement in several aspects of my body. The main adaption we're interested in is the ability to use the aerobic (fat burning) system. Because I avoid training above my lactic threshold, my fat burning enzymes began to improve.

I was now able to produce more energy from fat because I had trained in such a way as to command my body to produce more fat burning enzymes. The more of these enzymes we have, the quicker our body is able to produce energy from fat cells without having to tap into the glycolytic system. Of course there were other adaptations that took place during the training that allowed me to improve.

Most people's idea of progress with running is simply based on how far you can run within a given time. This usually means running hard and raising your heart rate to achieve this. Your body will adapt in many ways in order to achieve this, but since your main focus is to burn fat and to do so without having to workout, this method doesn't really lend itself here.

If you're vaguely interested in running or just want to do this experiment for yourself, I highly suggest it. As I've stated throughout this book, it's one thing to theorize, it's another to experience it for yourself. By using a heart rate monitor and distance tracker on your phone, you can see the results in action.

If you have zero interest in running, that's cool too. Even just going out for a brisk walk will begin to train your fat burning enzymes. You don't need to go all out by getting a heart rate monitor, tracking your runs, or training for your first 10km race.

There are a multitude of benefits to walking outdoors, especially in nature, that go beyond losing weight. Nature walks can help you enhance your mood, disconnect from the world, and even improve your sleep.

Beyond Fat Loss - Grounding Yourself

You may have heard the term grounding or earthing, but what does that mean? It simply means connecting to the earth. There are several ways you can do this. Walking barefoot, going to the beach, using an earthing mat, or even just placing your hand on the ground or a tree.

Humans are in a unique situation as we have removed ourselves from our natural ecosystem and substituted it with an artificial one. Climate control, soft beds, clothes, and shoes separate us from the animal world. But all of these creature comforts weaken our body as important biological triggers like hot/cold, famine/feast, and fight/flight have been taken from us.

You don't see any other animal on the planet separating itself from the earth the way humans do. Grounding is important for many reasons beyond just the physical and into mental, spiritual and emotional. These can be experienced once you start grounding and tuning into your body.

But what is happening on a physical level? Much like when you plug an appliance into the wall, and there is a port for the machine to "ground" and discharge an overload of electricity, us humans have a similar mechanism. When we touch the earth, we discharge energy that is not good for us.

When your body suffers from inflammation of any kind, free radicals tend to be created. If you've ever heard of antioxidants, you'll be interested in knowing that grounding is an amazing source of antioxidants. Without getting overly complicated, free radicals are atoms that have lost an electron in their outer shell, causing them to become unstable. This instability creates chaos in our bodies.

Our bodies want stable and reliable atoms. That's where antioxidants come in. Antioxidants donate their electrons to our atoms, allowing the outer shell to become complete and stable. The surface of the Earth is covered with a limitless supply of electrons that are waiting to join your body, reduce inflammation, and create stable atoms. Yet, as a species, we opt to live indoors, wear rubber shoes, and separate ourselves from the wild. Many people spend almost no time in nature or touching the Earth.

Think back to the last time you were at the beach. For most people, this is the only time they really get to ground. Most people go to the beach when they're on vacation. What happens after you spend a few hours there? Most likely, you feel tired and sleepy. I have a theory that may explain why that is.

During our daily life of work, family, and taking care of ourselves, we leave very little time in a stress-free environment to allow our bodies to recover properly. We are constantly in Go-Go-Go mode which leaves us feeling wired and tired.

When you go on vacation, relax, and ground through the beach, your body is finally allowed to fully go into parasympathetic mode (recovery/repair mode). Your body is so excited to go into this mode that it transfers its resources into healing your body. You might notice that the first few days you feel a little more tired than usual. After a week of being in this relaxed and stress-free state, your body has done a lot of healing and you feel revitalized.

Walking in nature daily can help you access this healing effect and make it part of your lifestyle. Not only do you get anti-oxidants if you choose to walk barefoot or simply put your hand on a tree, you also get a sense of peace that is hard to find by just chilling out and watching Netflix.

Bridge the Gap

1. The best time to walk is anytime you're actually willing to go. The second best is to start your morning off with a walk. Avoid eating beforehand to help tap into your fat stores more easily. A quick 10-15 minute walk is all you need to start your day off on the right foot.

2. If you have a fitness device or phone that can track your activity levels, use that to gauge yourself daily. If you're only hitting 2000-5000 steps a day, start to move the trend upward. See what your average is for week and then add 1000-2000 steps the next week. Gradually work up to 10,000-15,000 steps a day. Spread them throughout the day so you're staying active all day long.

3. Scheduling multiple walks throughout the day is ideal. They get you out of your chair, away from your screen, and increase your metabolism throughout the day. The easiest way to achieve this is to go for a 10 minute walk after each meal. Walking after a meal aids in digestion and helps reduce the amount of insulin released as some of the calories from your food are now going towards fueling your muscles instead of being stored as fat. This also had the added benefit of keeping your energy elevated after a meal instead of crashing afterwards.

4. Engage in an extended daily walk. A 30-60 minutes walk outside in nature without your phone is a fantastic way to turn on your fat burning system. Take this time to be alone with yourself. It's often in these moments that we have the greatest ideas and breakthroughs on what we are stuck on in work, relationships, and life.

5. If you do bring your phone, avoid listening to music. Instead, put on a motivational speech or lecture

on something relevant in your life. My personal recommendations are audio from Brian Tracey, Jim Rohn, and Paul Chek. Take this time as an opportunity to learn something new and engage in self-development.

6. Meditation while walking is another great option. Purposefully walking slower, focusing on deep breathing, and even counting your breaths are good options to keep you mindful and present.

7. When you go out anywhere (shopping, work, etc.) park in the furthest possible spot. This adds to your walking time without having to dedicate a specific time slot to it. Likewise, you can make it a rule that you must take the stairs anytime they are available instead of an elevator or escalators.

8. If you can walk or bike to work, stores, or friends, start to incorporate that into your routine. Instead of burning gasoline, burn your fat stores to get you from point A to point B. It's cheaper and better for you.

#7 RELAX, TAKE IT EASY

"One of the best pieces of advice I ever got was from a horse master. He told me to go slow in order to go fast. I think that applies to everything in life. We live as though there aren't enough hours in the day but if we do each thing calmly and carefully we will get it done quicker and with much less stress."

- Viggo Mortensen

2016 was one of the most stressful years of my life. Different pressures from all directions of my life had me feeling overwhelmed, anxious, depressed and as if I had no space to take care of myself. Alongside being a full-time student, I worked as a licensed realtor, a personal trainer, helping my parents with their business, creating online products, and running bootcamps outside of my local gym.

Video games helped me feel a semblance of happiness and allowed me to escape my reality. Much like a smoker that uses a cigarette to relax throughout the day, I was playing anytime I didn't have to engage with my responsibilities. Obviously this wasn't really helping me solve my problems. It was a band aid that kept me from being able to destress and assess my lifestyle.

Although I thought playing video games was relaxing, it was just another stimulus to my already overstimulated body and it ate into my sleep. What we perceive as relaxing is often a psychological release versus true relaxation. Doing something like playing a video game, watching a movie, or socializing can seem relaxing, but it doesn't fully allow your nervous system to rest and recover.

Temporarily removing all stimuli from your perception is the ideal way to allow your body to relax. Learning to truly let your body rest and recover is key to success in weight loss. Whether it's through meditating, walking in nature, or just laying in bed, take some time for yourself to remove external stimuli and just be with yourself. It's simple to say but not always easy to do. This section is dedicated to helping you relax and relieve stress.

Stress

Stress is a part of life that cannot be avoided. Learning to work with it is going to be critical for leading a healthy life and maintaining your weight goals. There are two types of stress a human can go through. Distress and Eustress. It's important to distinguish between the two as you want to minimize distress and optimize eustress.

Distress will cause damage to you, accelerating aging and may lead to physical, mental, emotional, and spiritual pain. Physical distress comes through as damage which your body has a hard time recovering from, leading to chronic pains. Repetitive or one-off injuries that are not dealt with properly can cause a lifetime of problems.

Some examples of physical distress would be eating bad food, being dehydrated, getting injured, not sleeping well, and having poor posture throughout the day. Distress can show up emotionally as well when your relationships aren't working out, you worry about the future, school isn't going well, work isn't going well or your finances are failing to name a few.

Eustress on the other hand, is seen as stress, you put yourself through that in the short term it is uncomfortable but in the long term it is beneficial. When you engage in something like fasting, working out, or going out into the cold you are triggering stress responses in your body.

These types of actions induce what is known as a hormetic response. Hormetic stressors, such as working out, are considered acute and controlled acts that help stimulate healthy adaptive responses that the body thrives on. It's about finding the optimal dose to produce the effect you want. Not too much but not too little.

Remember, we were designed to be out in the wild. Nature has many natural stressors that are good for us when exposed to them for a limited time. Running away from predators and hunting helped to keep our muscles and bones strong by providing a stimulus.

There is a concept known as Wolff's law which states the bones will adapt to the loads under which they are put. If you don't put stress on your bones, they will weaken and become brittle. If you lift weights, the stress of your muscles pulling on the bones will force them to grow stronger. Your body adapts to the demands you put on it, and if you don't provide sources of eustress, there is no reason for it to improve or to maintain what it already has.

If we take the opposite approach, we can consider how many people live sedentary lifestyles where they provide very limited amounts of stimulation to their muscles. This causes strength, muscle mass, and bone density to decrease. In order to grow and improve yourself, you need to provide a stimulus.

Understand that in order for a hormetic effect to occur, you need the right amount of stimulus. You wouldn't spend 8 hours in a gym everyday, that's overkill and will lead to negative results because you're not giving your body time to recover. 1 hour a day a few times a week is plenty.

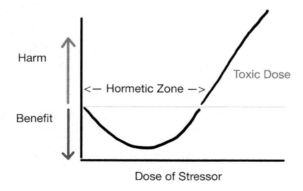

Be smart about this. Start gradually and build up. If you were to try squatting 500lbs on your first day in the gym, your muscles and bones would shatter. That's why I've provided the steps for you to bridge the gap in these habits and a plethora of tools so your body and mind can adapt through consistent progress rather than be shocked from short term and extreme efforts.

The goal is to start incorporating more hormetic (eustress) activities along with practices that help reduce the negative effects of distress by calming your mind and nervous system.

Stress is Holding You Back

Distress stops the repair and recovery functions of your body. When you're stressed, your body's blood delivery system changes. It constricts and limits the blood vessels that go towards your organs and digestive system in order to funnel the blood to the muscles.

You have about 100,000km of blood vessels. Your body has the ability to reduce and increase blood flow into certain regions. When your body receives the stress signal, it thinks that you are in an emergency situation and nutrients need to be brought to the muscles in order to survive.

If you've ever eaten a meal and then tried playing a sport, working out, or running, you've likely noticed that heavy feeling in your gut. That's your stomach shutting down in order to provide more energy to your muscles. This occurs even if you're not doing physical activity. Stress diverts resources away from vital organs and digestive function.

Distress also stops your creativity and imagination. As Paul Chek says, "If you're being chased by a lion, you don't throw in a cartwheel." When you're under constant stress it makes it difficult to be creative and engage with the processes that will ultimately change your life. Survival mode leads to tunnel vision, making it hard to see alternative ways of living.

All stress summates in your body. Imagine having one big bucket that represents the amount of stress your body can handle. All the stress you experience goes into that one bucket. Once you reach the limit and it starts to overflow, your body is no longer capable of recovering fast enough from the stress and you begin to experience acute and chronic problems.

Stress comes from every part of your life. Your relationships, work, food intake, sleep, and even a lack of clarity in life can all add up to overfill your stress bucket. That's why the first activity you do in this book is to become clear on your goals and purpose. So that you can infuse love and motivation into the activities you deem necessary for you to live a happy and healthy life.

I've seen countless people walk into the gym who work 10+ hours a day, don't sleep, don't eat or hydrate well, and are red-lining their life on all fronts. Then they proceed to do an intense, hour-long workout, which they think is serving them when in reality they are putting more stress into an already overflowing bucket.

If you're experiencing this level of stress and are still trying to fit more into your life, I'm here to invite you into another way. Instead of hammering out more, start by removing the things that don't align and don't serve you. Instead of an intense workout, go for a walk, stretch, or do some yoga.

The following breathing and meditation techniques will help to scoop stress out of your bucket. These are here to make your life easier. You don't need to meditate for 30 minutes right off the bat. Make small commitments of 2-5 minutes throughout the day to engage with these practices and build from there.

A major mistake I see in people who repeatedly fail to achieve their goals is that they pick goals that are far beyond what they've achieved in the past. If you've previously been able to meditate for 20 minutes consistently, start with 50% of that by committing to 10 minutes.

The dark side of this is when people who have never been able to meditate or engage in any breathing practice for more than 2 minutes decide to commit to 20 minutes a day. This is like my running example in the beginning of the book. If you've never run a marathon before, don't start with that as your first goal.

Breathe

What's the most important nutrient in your body? In order to answer this, you have to consider what would cause you to die the fastest if you ran out of it. You can go months without food if you've got enough fat reserves. You can go multiple days without water. The number one nutrient you can't survive more than minutes without is oxygen. This is the most vital substance you can pull into your body yet 99% of people neglect focusing on adequate oxygen intake.

The average person breathes roughly 25,000x/day. Unfortunately they also tend to breathe improperly. There are a few mechanisms that you are likely not doing correctly that are severely hampering your ability to lose weight and live a life full of energy and vibrance.

When you combine food, water, and oxygen you can create an energy surplus in your body that makes you feel alive. When you lack good food, hydration, and air you force your body to run on fumes. When you can elevate your vitality and bring excitement to your life through your breath, then you begin to do more than just lose weight. You begin to grab life by the horns.

Mouth Breathers

Mouth breathing is a problem that many people unknowingly suffer from. You want to do your best to avoid breathing through your mouth. Instead, you should focus on breathing through your nose, which stimulates your parasympathetic nervous system, which triggers rest and relaxation.

Mouth breathing triggers a sympathetic nervous response,

putting you into fight or flight mode. It also engages what's known as accessory breathing muscles in your neck and rib cage. These muscles are meant to be used in short bursts to help increase your breathing if you're attacking or being attacked.

When you engage these small accessory muscles to the exclusion of the primary muscle of respiration, namely the diaphragm, you are now causing an excessive demand 25,000x a day. This leads to small muscles doing repetitive work all day leading to chronic neck and shoulder pain due to the overuse of these accessory muscles.

When you breathe through your nose, focus on keeping your tongue gently pressed against the roof of your mouth, behind your front top teeth. This mechanism works much like a seatbelt. By pressing your tongue up, you create an anchor point for the flexor (front) muscles of your neck, allowing you to stabilize your head much more effectively.

According to Chinese medicine, putting your tongue on the roof of your mouth works to connect the Ren (conception) vessel with the Du (governing) vessel. This connection between two vital circuits in your body helps promote the flow of qi and life force energy.

Nose breathing is so important that there are even advanced devices that help you achieve optimal sleep at night. Of course, I'm talking about using tape over your mouth to ensure you're not breathing improperly all night. There are a lot of tapes out there, but I'd recommend using something specific for the task as you don't want to use regular masking tape.

Diaphragmatic Breathing

Alongside nose breathing, you will need to focus on engaging your diaphragm. The diaphragm is a large muscle that cuts across the middle of your torso. When this muscle contracts, it helps to expand your lungs so air can come in. The diaphragm works by creating negative pressure in your lungs by expanding them. When they expand, the pressure inside them is reduced, causing air from the outside (which is at a higher pressure) to come into your lungs.

Taking your diaphragm through a full range of motion also creates a pumping effect for your organs and spine. When you fully breathe in, your belly expands and your organs move around. When your diaphragm isn't fully engaged, your organs stay stagnant. You need a pumping movement to aid with the removal of waste and to bring in nutrients.

Deep diaphragmatic breathing also works to pump CSF (cerebral spinal fluid) through your brain. When you exhale, your spinal curvature (cervical, thoracic, and lumber) increases, allowing CSF to move downward. When you inhale, your spinal curvature decreases, thus forcing the CSF upwards into your brain.

Many mechanisms go awry when you don't use your diaphragm. If CSF isn't circulating well, you can experience brain fog, fatigue, and a lack of creativity. CSF helps to bring in nutrients and remove waste from your brain. The media and Hollywood tend to teach us to value a smaller waist and therefore constantly suck the belly inwards to create this illusion. Allowing your belly to move naturally is critical to good health.

Deep Breaths

The final mechanism you're likely unaware of is the amount of oxygen you take in per breath. Most people only use 1/7 of their lung capacity during normal breathing. A lightbulb should be going off in your head right now. You're probably working at 1/7 your energy capacity if you're only using 14% of your lungs' capacity.

Put another way, you're reducing your metabolism because you're limiting your fat burning system by not allowing enough oxygen to enter. Oxygen is the fuel for many life processes, the more you can get in you, generally speaking, the better your will function. If you're only breathing at 14% or reduced capacity, you're likely not engaging in nose or diaphragmatic breathing.

Utilizing nose, diaphragmatic, and full depth breathing through the techniques you're about to learn will do wonders for de-stressing your body and giving it permission to let go of the fat it's been holding on to due to stress. Emptying your stress bucket through breathing is one of the simplest and cheapest things you can do for your health.

But hold on, do you know what triggers your body to take in a breath? Most people would say that a lack of oxygen signals your brain to send the message to breath. However, it's the buildup of CO_2 (carbon dioxide) that triggers breathing. As CO_2 builds up, your blood becomes more and more acidic.

Your blood needs to stay within a very narrow window of acidity or else all hell breaks loose. This is around a pH of 7.4. Your natural metabolism and consumption of oxygen causes CO_2 to be released constantly. When you engage in physical activity, your muscles produce much more CO_2 causing your heart rate and breathing rate to increase in order to deal with the excess CO_2.

When you try to hold your breath, it's not the fact that you're using up oxygen that triggers the urge to breathe. It's the buildup of CO_2 because you are no longer removing it from your blood. As CO_2 builds up, your diaphragm begins to spasm until you eventually give in and take a breath.

The buildup of CO_2 serves a very important purpose beyond triggering you to breathe. As CO_2 builds up, it causes oxygen to more readily dissociate from the hemoglobin that binds it to red blood cells. Thus, leaving more oxygen for your tissues to use.

To make this simple, imagine a RBC (red blood cell) with 4 ports to hold oxygen. When it leaves your lungs and is pumped out by your heart, it has 4 oxygen molecules attached to it. In order for your muscles, organs, and tissues to get the oxygen,

RBC has to release it along its journey through your arteries.

RBCs have a certain affinity for oxygen. If they didn't, they wouldn't be able to hold onto them as they went through your lungs. When there is a higher concentration of CO_2 in your blood, it makes it much easier for your RBC to release the oxygen molecules vs a lower CO_2 concentration.

If you can get more oxygen into your tissues, they can produce more energy for themselves and ultimately for you. Keep this in mind as we now go into techniques you can use to practice breathing and reduce the load in your stress bucket. You want to be able to increase your capacity to comfortably handle more CO_2 so that more oxygen can be delivered to your tissues.

As you practice breathing techniques and maintain awareness of the importance of CO_2, you will start to increase your CO_2 threshold. The threshold is where you initially start to feel the need to breathe. Through practice, you can elevate your threshold thus allowing you to seamlessly have more CO_2 in your bloodstream leading to greater oxygen utilization.

You will likely have a low threshold when you start, making it harder to hold your breath and do some of the breathing exercises. Fear not, as you train yourself to push yourself into some discomfort, your CO_2 threshold will increase, meaning that your breathing will naturally slow down during the day.

Slower breathing will help calm your nervous system and will keep more CO_2 in your system. Remember, do your best to breathe through your nose, engage your diaphragm, and take fuller breaths throughout the day, not just during practice.

One small caveat. There are, of course, exceptions to the rules. There will always be times and techniques where breathing through your mouth will be preferred and smaller breaths will be used. Again, don't be dogmatic in your methods. See what each technique does for you and then decide if you want to keep it.

Breathing Techniques

As you go through these techniques, stop after you read each one and try it right away. See how your body feels about it and decide if you like it and want to keep practicing it. There is no sense in reading through a bunch of techniques and being bogged down after trying to remember what's what. You will get the best results by immediately implementing these and practicing them right away.

As Bruce Lee said, "I don't fear the man who can throw 10,000 different kicks. I fear the man who has thrown one kick 10,000 times". The more you practice with a technique, the more it will do for you. You don't need 20 practices. You only need 1-3 that are effective for you.

Diaphragm Activation

The first thing you need to establish is how to activate and engage your diaphragm. There are 3 techniques we will use for this. Use whichever one gets you the best connection to your diaphragm. Try all three and continue practicing the one that gets you the best result.

<u>Your Two Hands</u>

1. While sitting or laying down, place one hand over your belly button and the other one over your chest.

2. Exhale and gently draw your belly button towards your spine. This causes your hand to move as well.

3. Inhale and expand your belly into your hand, moving your belly button away from your spine.

4. As you inhale, the first ⅔ will come from your belly and the last third comes from your chest.

5. Repeat for 2-5 minutes

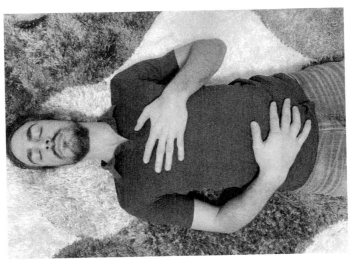

Hands are used as visual/tactile feedback. Your belly rising indicates that your diaphragm is contracting. As the belly falls, your diaphragm is relaxing. Prioritize your belly moving before your chest to avoid overloading your neck muscles.

Crocodile Breath

1. Lay on your chest on a soft floor. Keep your head in a neutral position with your fingers stacked on top of each other and use them as a cushion for your forehead.

2. Exhale and gently draw your belly button towards your spine, as If you're trying to take your belly button off the floor.

3. There is no need to lift your belly from the floor. Do not engage your hips or cheat this movement. You want to isolate it as much as possible.

4. Inhale and expand your belly into the floor as if you're trying to move past it.

5. The first ⅔ of your breath comes from the belly rising and the final third comes from your chest.

6. Repeat for 2-5 minutes

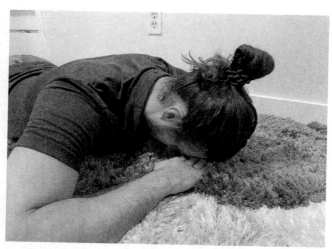

Water Bottle

1. Lay on your back and put a water bottle on your belly. This should not be a heavy bottle but should still have some weight so you can get feedback.

2. Exhale and gently draw the belly button towards the spine. The water bottle will move closer to the floor.

3. Inhaling with the aim of expanding your belly and water bottle upwards.

4. The first ⅔ of the breath comes from the belly and the final third comes from the chest.

5. Repeat for 2-5 minutes.

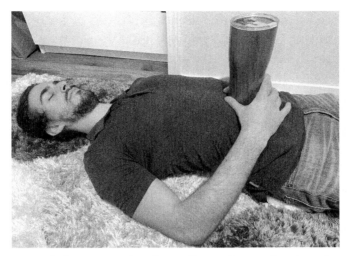

Each one of these can be done for a few minutes throughout the day. Once you figure out how to engage your diaphragm properly and take full deep breaths that start from the belly and finish in the chest, you won't need these 3 exercises.

These 3 practices will help you create a connection with your diaphragm and will lead to the positive results discussed previously. However, we want to start making this part of your every waking moment and not just a practice you do for 5 minutes a day.

The goal of these exercises is to move beyond them. With a little bit of practice, you will be able to take a functional breath without needing the feedback of the floor, a water bottle or your hands. Bringing awareness to your breath throughout the day can be done in so many different ways. Here are the two main ways I recommend, but by all means do whatever you need to do to remember to take full breaths throughout the day.

1) Set an Alarm

Every hour on the hour from 9am-5pm, set an alarm to go off. Commit to taking anywhere from 3-10 deep breaths when the alarms go off.

2) Use a String

Tie a string around your waist. It should be snug but not too tight. Having this string here will give you constant feedback. You can breathe into the string to encourage proper form. This is not forever. This is just to help reset your breathing patterns until proper breathing becomes unconscious for you.

Breathing Practices

You wouldn't start making weapons after you get into a war. You want to have your weapons ready for when war happens. Likewise, if you try using these techniques only when you're under stress, you are undercutting your results. Practicing these techniques when you're in a calm state of mind will help you cultivate them so they will better serve you when you're under stress as well.

Pick a few techniques and train them consistently. Even having just one of these down well will do wonders. You don't need to start off by doing all of them. Set a timer and make a commitment to doing at least one of these daily for 2 minutes. Build up by doing them a few times throughout the day and then continue to improve by adding more time during each session.

<u>4 in, 2 out</u>

1. Inhale for 4 seconds.
2. Gently exhale for 2 seconds.
3. Repeat

Optional - Increase the time as you become more comfortable. For example, 6s in, 3s out. 8s in, 4s out etc.

Simply put, you are inhaling twice as long as you are exhaling. You can use metronome for external feedback. Start with 60 beats per minute such that every second the metronome makes a sound. If you decrease the beats to 50, you will make the exercise harder.

I personally like putting my hand on my chest and using my heartbeat instead of the metronome. This allows me to focus inward into my heart rather than outward. Choose whatever serves you best. Do not release too much air on the exhale. You are not trying to empty your lungs on this one. This technique will help you gently become accustomed to building up CO_2 in your blood and improving your threshold.

4x4 Breath

1. Inhale for 4s
2. Hold your breath for 4s
3. Exhale for 4s
4. Hold for 4s
5. Repeat

This style of breathing helps to relax your nervous system and will help you deal with stress, anxiety, worry, and overwhelming situations. It is a technique that military soldiers are taught to use to calm themselves down before storming a building or entering a dangerous situation.

Complete Breath

1. Inhale starting from your belly, aiming to fill the lowest lobes of your lungs
2. Continue inhaling, aiming to fill and expand the middle of your chest.
3. At the peak of your inhale, shrug your shoulders to maximize the lung space in your upper rib cage.
4. Exhale and release all the air.

The goal of this exercise is to use as much of your lung capacity as possible. Allow yourself to focus inwards on your lungs so that you can fill every part of it. This will help you increase your lung usage from 1/7th their capacity. You will experience a surge of energy (possibly heat as well) and a strong connection to your body if you follow through with this.

Cleansing Breath

1. Kneel down with an upright torso

2. Inhale and hold for 7s

3. Exhale in bursts by snapping your belly button towards your spine

4. Hinge at your waist and bring your head towards the floor as you exhale

5. Fully empty your lungs to the best of your ability while in a folded position

6. Inhale and raise yourself back up

7. Repeat

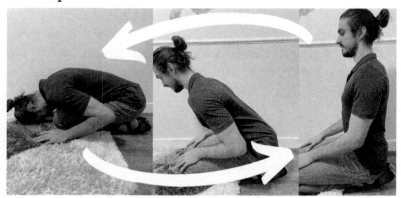

Your lungs share the same entrance and exit. With shallow breaths and even with deeper, more focused breaths, stagnant air gets trapped. By doing the cleansing breaths, you're able to remove stale air from all corners of your lungs. This exercise also helps to strengthen the muscles of exhalation.

Slow Breathing

1. Inhale as slowly and as continuously as you can

2. Hold your breath at the peak for as long as you feel comfortable

3. Exhale as slowly and continuously as you can

4. Hold your breath as long as you feel comfortable

5. Repeat

Set a timer. Your goal is to take the least amount of breath possible using this technique during this time period. This takes a lot of focus and effort but can produce a peaceful state of mind while helping you deal with stress. Concentrating on your breath to this level keeps you present and stops you from wandering into the past and future.

Breath holds (Wim Hof style)

1. Complete 30-50 exaggerated breaths

    a. Deep full inhales with a relaxed and shallow exhale

    b. Getting tingles in your body is normal

    c. You may feel a little dizzy or lightheaded as well

2. On the final breath, take a full inhalation and a relaxed exhale before starting a breath hold.

3. Time your hold.

4. When you need to, slowly exhale your air and hold for 15s

5. Inhale fully and hold for at least 15s.

6. Repeat

Wim Hof breathing has become extremely popular and there are lots of resources that exist for this method. It is often combined with cold exposure for a powerful nervous system stimulation.

Breath holds on Empty

1. Complete 30-50 exaggerated breaths

    a. Deep full inhales with a relaxed and shallow exhale

    b. Getting tingles in your body is normal

    c. You may feel a little dizzy or lightheaded as well

2. On the final breath, take a full inhalation and a full exhalation, removing as much air as you feel comfortable. You want to hold your breath without having too much air in your lungs

3. Time your hold.

4. When you need to, take a big inhalation and continue to hold your breath.

5. Release your breath hold when you can no longer maintain it

6. Repeat

Unlike previous exercises, this method allows you to retain the CO_2 you've built up and continue your breath hold by taking in a big breath after you can no longer hold on empty. This allows you to continue to accumulate CO_2 and improve your tolerance to it.

<u>Walking breath holds</u>

1. As you walk, bring attention to your breath.

2. Take a few calm, not exaggerated breaths with focused attention

3. When ready, inhale and then exhale such that you're at about half your lung capacity

4. Hold your breath and count how many steps you travel

5. Do not push past the urge to breathe. Inhale when holding your breath becomes uncomfortable

6. When you inhale, take no more than 3 breaths to restore your breathing pattern. You should not be gasping for air.

7. Repeat again when you're ready

This is a technique I learned from the book *"The oxygen advantage"* by Patrick McKeown. I highly recommend this book.

No one should be able to tell that you're doing this exercise from start to finish. These breath holds are subtle and help to improve your CO_2 threshold. Patrick's book is where I learned about the CO_2 threshold theory and it has many more exercises on improving your breathing.

<u>Othership</u>

Othership is the best app I've used for breathing exercises. They have a wide variety of styles but my favorite are the energizing tracks. Your breathing is cued and synced to uplifting music that makes breath work fun and engaging. They usually include breath holds and a buffet of different breathing techniques for whatever needs you may have.

Meditation

The word meditation makes some people happy while it instills fear in others. If you have never been able to meditate for more than 30 seconds in your life, I have good news for you. There is a very clear reason for this, and I have an extremely straightforward way to overcome it.

The problem with meditation is that no one teaches you the ABCs of meditating. They always give you a specific task like "focus on your breath" or imagine a white light in your chest, but they don't give you the tools to properly achieve and follow the meditation.

Through the practice of something known as contemplative meditation, you will learn the ABCs of meditation. You will be able to calm your mind and focus not only on the meditation at hand but rather, you will see improvements in your daily life.

Contemplative meditation is something I learned from my friend Michael Holt. After practising this, my understanding of meditation changed. Once you get this, you can apply it to any meditation with great success.

Contemplative Meditation

You are going to focus on the development of 3 key characteristics through contemplative meditation.

1. Concentration

The mental effort you direct toward whatever you're working on or learning in the moment

2. Sensory Clarity

The ability to track your sensory experience (what you are seeing, hearing, feeling, etc.) in real time.

3. Equanimity

Mental calmness, composure, and evenness of temper, especially in a difficult situation.

All 3 are important to develop and can be worked on together, however, we will start with a focus on concentration. Without concentration power, you can sit in "meditation" for an hour but if your mind is wandering and thinking about something else, the impact of meditation is reduced.

Concentration is a master skill that applies to everything in your life. Concentration grants the ability to stay in the present instead of unconsciously drifting into the future or past. In this way, you can get more out of life by living in the present instead of spending your time in the future or past.

Frustration from meditation may arise due to its subjective nature. Things like "focus on your breath" or "empty your mind" are hard to see and track progress in. That's why we are going to build your concentration from the ground up, using objective measures and ways to track your progress.

The brain is like a muscle, so we will be treating meditation like going to the gym. Sets and reps will be tracked to see progress over time. If you want to improve your focus and concentration power, you need to train it like anything else.

1) Concentration

To improve concentration, your goal will be to count your inhales and exhales with 100% accuracy for a given time period or number of sets. As your concentration improves and your accuracy stays at 100%, you can increase the time period, sets or change the counting method to make it more challenging.

The Rules:

1. Inhales occur on **odd** numbers (1,3,5,7)

2. Exhales occur on **even** numbers (2,4,6,8)

3. Once you get to 8, you go back to 1

If, at any given point, you don't know with 100% certainty which breath number you are on, you have failed the set and must restart.

If you're on the 5th count (which should be an inhale), but you're exhaling, you know you've lost track and should restart.

If you count beyond 8, you have lost track and must restart.

The slower you breathe, the more challenging this will be.

1. Inhale = 1
2. Exhale = 2
3. Inhale = 3
4. Exhale = 4
5. Inhale = 5
6. Exhale = 6
7. Inhale = 7
8. Exhale = 8
9. Repeat starting at 1

You can start by doing sets of 30 seconds for this. 30 seconds will likely not be long enough time to get to 8 counts. That's ok. If you only get to 4 or 5 that is perfectly acceptable, there is no expectation to complete all the breaths within 30 seconds.

If 30 seconds is too easy, bump it up to 45 seconds or 60 seconds. I recommend using a stopwatch or timer for your initial practices. Once you become proficient with 2 minutes of straight concentration, you can perform your practice without a timer if you so choose. Completing a full count of 8 would equal one set. You can then make your goal to complete 3-5 sets straight instead of aiming for 2-5 minutes straight. Once that becomes easy, you can change the rules of counting.

For example, instead of resetting back to 1 after you finished your 8 count, you can inhale and count 7, then exhale and count 6. You are now counting both up and down. The challenge comes when, for instance, you are inhaling on the count of 5 and have to remember if you are counting up to 6 or counting down to 4 on the next breath.

If, when you start, you can only complete 1 set or 45 seconds without losing your concentration, you now have an objective starting point. Much like someone who can only do 3 push ups when they start working out. After a few days or weeks of consistent practice, your concentration ability should drastically increase. You will be able to complete 3-5 sets straight without losing your position where previously you might have barely completed one set.

This would lead to you increasing your concentration power as objectively as someone who started at 3 push ups and can now do 20 push ups. I would, pun intended, focus on this exercise as your primary form of meditation at the beginning. Once your newly acquired ability to focus has been trained, move onto the sensory aspect and equanimity portions of contemplative meditation.

Make a commitment to do 3-5 successful sets per day or 5 minutes of total time. They can be in a row or spread out through the day. If you can do 5 minutes of perfectly concentrated breathing and counting, you will possess a concentration power that few people have.

With this concentration power you will be able to maximize your time spent doing other meditations as you will be able to do them instead of having your mind wander off. Also, this will help cultivate your ability to stay in the present moment and not let your mind pull you into the future or past.

2) Sensory Clarity

The ability to track your sensory experience (what you are seeing, hearing, thinking, etc.) in real time is critical for being able to tune into your body and stay in the present. When I first learned this, I didn't really understand the gold that was hidden behind the simple exercise. If you can understand this, you can know what it means to live in the present moment.

Sensory clarity is what I would consider a practice of presence and mindfulness. It directs your mind to focus on bodily sensations you're currently experiencing. By bringing attention to this, you stop your mind from wandering into the past and into the future.

There are three main aspects of this that you will be focusing on: seeing, hearing, and feeling. Each of these will be broken down into their own practice and then brought together. Of course there are also the sense of smell and taste which this practice can extend to but we will not be addressing in this book.

Each of these 3 aspects has 2 dimensions. The external and internal. For example, you can have your eyes open and see a book, a table, and a phone. If you close your eyes, you can visualize a book, a table, and a phone. One is happening objectively in the external world and one is happening subjectively in your internal field of view.

When it comes to the sense of feeling, the external and internal stimuli equally apply. Externally, you may feel your clothes on your skin, your butt in a chair, the temperature, an itch, or pressure coming from a massage. Internally, you may feel stressed, anxious, happy, sad, excited, or you may be feeling a sensation of tightness or pain in a certain region.

Training your sensory clarity is about paying attention to, identifying, and then releasing your attention from the stimulus. Rather than getting drawn into one sensation or story, you want to recognize when it grabs your attention and then let it go, allowing for the next moment to continue to be in the present.

There are three levels to this practice. The first level takes place in the dedicated time and space you choose to do your meditation. The second level is bringing the practice into your daily life by bringing the same degree of awareness to your waking activities. Level three is the practice of staying present throughout the day in all three senses. You will better understand this as we go through the exercises.

Seeing

You can practice this with your eyes open during the first half and with your eyes closed during the second half. Set a timer for 2-5 minutes and focus your attention on what you see in front of you. If an object captures your attention with your eyes open, simply name it. You can state the color, shape, size, etc. Then allow the next visual stimulus to become the center of your focus.

Next, you will close your eyes and pay attention to what comes up in your visual field. You do not need to use your imagination and make things appear. Simply sit in stillness with your focus on what you see in your mind's eye. Once something comes up, acknowledge that you see it and then release it.

Do not allow your brain to wander off into a visual story or through the voices in your head. Your goal is to solely concentrate on your visual sense in order to hone it and bring you into the present.

Through this, you are practicing staying in the present moment and seeing what's in front of you. How many times have you walked or driven by the same location yet not really seen it? One day you ask yourself "is this new or has it always been there?". Most of us are getting from point A to B stuck in our heads, living in the past or future rather than paying attention to the present stimulus that's occurring before us.

By practicing this first in a meditation setting, you are able to build the foundations. When you bring it into your walks, talks, or even while doing the dishes you are enlivening the practice and keeping yourself in the present.If you want to stress yourself out and worry, thinking about the future or the past will usually do the job. If you want to live in peace and harmony, spending more time in the present is often a good start.

Hearing

To practice this, set aside 2-5 minutes of dedicated time during the day. You can close your eyes or keep them open. Being outside will allow for more external stimulus. Try both inside and outside to see which you prefer. As an external sound captures your attention, tune into it for a moment, acknowledge that you heard it, and then let it go. Allow your focus to stay in the present and not linger on anything.

As an internal sound or voice captures your attention, tune into it for a moment, acknowledge it, and then let it go. Do not allow yourself to be pulled into a dialogue or story. This is what draws you out of the present moment. It is often internal voices, sometimes your own or someone else's, that drag us into the past and future. This is where anxiety and worry reside.

Practice allowing stimulation to catch your present attention, be aware that it is doing so, and then let it go.

Feeling

The practice of feeling is twofold. Set aside 2-5 minutes for this. You can spend the first half of the exercise focusing on what you feel externally. The sensation of your pants, your shirt, your hair, the wind, an itch, the pressure from the ground, and the temperature. During the second half of your practice, you will focus on what you feel internally. This can sound familiar to something called a body scan, but it's important to avoid doing that here. Your aim is to pay attention to any sensation that arises inside you.

Give your body permission to release and notice any sensations, feelings or emotions that arise. Make a note of the location where you feel it. Whether it's in your head, neck, shoulder, chest, abdomen, hips or legs. Notice it, acknowledge it, and release it to allow for the next sensation to occur without being attached to a past experience.

The ability to tune into one's feelings and emotions is becoming increasingly rare in Western society. We are taught to be logical, take painkillers and have antidepressants distributed to us before lifestyle therapies and interventions are used. We are often hypnotized into separating from our bodies and transporting our minds into electronic devices.

All of these act as distractions and numb us from seeing the truth that our bodies are so frantically trying to tell our minds. There are so many external forces fighting for our attention that it becomes difficult to turn down the noise and feel into what really matters.

Emotions and feelings are powerful forces that must be heard. There are reasons why you feel what you feel. By acknowledging and listening to the feeling, we allow it to pass through and out of us. We also get to learn the lessons they bring with them.

In Chinese Medicine, it is excess emotions that are not allowed to flow that cause internal diseases. There are no bad emotions. Western society creates the divide of good and bad while bringing shame to certain emotions and glory to others.

All emotions are important and are teachers for you. If you feel pain or sadness, perhaps there is a lesson for the future in how you can grow from what occurred. Far too many people shy away from feelings and emotions in retreat to the sanctuary of Netflix, alcohol, and Haagen-Dazs. This is where the following practice of contemplative meditation becomes relevant and important.

Sensory clarity in practice

Level one:

Do all of these practices at rest and with your full attention to it for 2-5 minutes. Allow your training in concentration to take over in order to keep focus during this task.

<u>Level two:</u>

Dedicate 15-30 minutes to each sense while you do daily activities. For example, as you cook your meal, you can focus on what you see for 15 minutes.

For example: I see a knife, I see a sink, I see my hands, I see meat. Do not be afraid to repeat items you see over and over again. That is simply what caught your present moment's attention. There is no need to avoid repetition. You are doing this so you can stay in the present moment with your activity instead of drifting off into the past or future. Practice this dedicated time with your hearing and feeling sensations as well. Perhaps you walk to work and can use that time for this dedicated practice. See how you feel during and once you get to your destination.

<u>Level three:</u>

Combine all three sensations into every aspect of your daily life. Staying present with these 3 senses throughout the day, anytime you remember, will be the ultimate practice that brings you in the present moment. This keeps you mindful, aware of your body, and helps you connect to yourself and others.

Consider adding smell and taste to level three practices. The exercise of mindful eating, which was discussed earlier in the book, can help enliven your sense of taste and smell. Engage these senses along with the previous 3 to make eating a full sensory experience.

3) Equanimity

Being able to hold mental calmness, composure, and evenness of temper, especially in a difficult situation is vital to living a balanced and healthy life. Equanimity is the ability to not be swayed by "good" or "bad" experiences. This will help you keep inner peace and make quality decisions in life.

The importance of equanimity becomes evident in three aspects of our lives. When we are alone, interacting with another person, or interacting with the world. Equanimity allows us to keep composure in the face of fear and excitement.

When you are alone, do you allow your feelings and emotions to dictate what you do? Do you tend to go towards that uncomfortable feeling inside you with an open and unrelenting mindset or does it scare you away into distracting yourself to avoid the void? When you practice equanimity, you accept anything that comes up in the present moment.

If you are interacting with someone, do you allow your feelings and emotions to control how you speak to that person? Can you listen and not be stirred outwardly as well as inwardly? Engaging with people in a reactionary manner tends to cause problems in relationships and breaks down communication. When you can be still and connect to your feelings without letting them take over, you can come to more solid resolutions with your spouse, friends, family, and business partners.

When it comes to applying equanimity towards the world, do you let factors that you have no control over infest your mind? Does watching the news, reading papers, and listening to your government cause your mood to shift and your peace of mind to fade?

Listening to your body is number one. Getting in touch with your feelings and not letting them persuade you into highs and lows is how you can maintain level composure. Equanimity is not just about staying calm in the face of bad news. It equally applies to good emotions and feelings as well.

Without equanimity towards the positive aspects in life, our vices and addictions start to take over. If you drink alcohol or party, can you avoid becoming attached to the good feelings they bring you? If you don't bring equanimity to the good things in your life it can lead you down the path of avoiding the bad and numbing with the good.

The practice of equanimity requires you to sit in the middle of your emotions without letting them take over you.

Presence and Mindfulness

You have just learned the ABCs of all meditation exercises. With practice and consistency, you can bring concentration, sensory clarity, and equanimity to any aspect of your life. This is a powerful skill to develop that will show up in all aspects of your life, not just while you're on a meditation cushion.

From now on, when you hear someone asking you to "be more present" or "mindful", this is what they're talking about. They want you to concentrate, be clear on what you see, hear, and feel, along with being in a state of equanimity instead of allowing your emotions to burst out of you.

You might at this point be wondering what all this has to do with weight loss. It has everything to do with weight loss. The way you interact with yourself, others, and the world has a massive impact on your ability to lose weight and be healthy.

If you can't concentrate, how do you expect to follow through with anything in this book? If you can't get clear on how your body feels and stay in the present moment, how are you going to change your future? Without conscious present moment effort, you will keep reliving your past, allowing it to dictate your future.

You cannot change your future with your past. Only your presence can change your future. If you can't engage with your feelings and emotions in a healthy manner, how do you expect to overcome negative and positive emotions that have dictated your behavior thus far?

I sincerely hope you understand the massive, life-changing benefits of contemplative meditation. Not only will it help with all the above, but it will also help reduce your stress levels, which as we've already discussed, will help you lose weight.

Physical Acts of Meditation

If sitting still and meditating isn't your cup of tea, I'd like to give you the opportunity to engage in meditation using more physical alternatives. As long as you're able to focus, tune into your body and stay on task these meditation practices will work well.

The old adage of "what's the best diet or exercise to do?" applies to meditation as well. The "best" meditation is the one you will do consistently. These are a few of my favorite ways to incorporate moving meditations into my practice.

Moving Stagnant Liver Qi

According to Chinese Medicine theory, unfulfilled desires cause stress. This stress transforms and can cause something known as LQS (liver qi stagnation). LQS is common in western society. The liver is responsible for the smooth flow of qi in your body. It influences the flow of all qi and can impact multiple organ systems. This shows up when you are under more stress than usual. The liver "attacks" other organs and impacts their functions.

People react to this differently. For some, their digestion is impacted. For others, they may get headaches and acne on their face. In other cases, skin issues may flair up when under stress, again showing a lack of smooth, free flowing liver qi.

My favorite exercise for moving the liver is a qigong move called liver tossing. It was taught to me by one of my professors and I have used it to great success. As a matter of fact, I use this exercise to help stimulate my flow of qi and creativity before I begin writing.

Liver Tossing

1. Stand tall with feet shoulder width apart.
2. Inhale and raise both arms out to the side up to shoulder height
3. Exhale and at the same time rotate your torso to the right

   - Your left hand will mimic an underhand throw in front and across your body towards the right side

   - Your right hand will swing behind your back towards the left

4. Inhale and reset to position in step 2
5. Exhale and repeat step 3 but this time go towards the left
6. Repeat for 2-5 minutes at a moderate pace

Avoid having stiff legs or muscles. As you "toss" in each direction, imagine negative energy being tossed away. Ensure you don't just let the energy out near yourself. You want to launch the negative energy away to maintain energetic hygiene in your area.

This meditation involves a lot of torso rotation which also helps to pump your organs and digestive system. Therefore, along with releasing negative energy and moving your liver qi, you are also improving your internal health by bringing more nutrients into your core and removing waste.

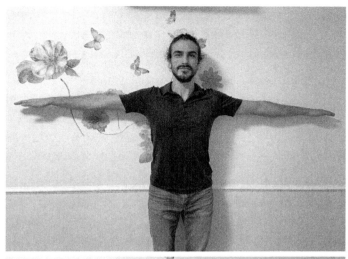

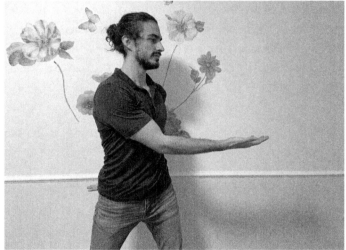

Another great way to stimulate the flow of qi in your body along with releasing any dense energies is to practice shaking.

Shaking

1. Stand with feet shoulder width apart
2. Slowly begin to shake your limbs and body.
3. You can do rhythmic shake forwards, side to side, or up and down.
4. Mix it up, don't get stuck.

Eventually, you want to feel as though someone or something else is shaking you. Allow your body to go on autopilot and shake itself in any way it wants to release.

This is a great way to move your qi as well as all the joints in your body. Your body needs movement in order to clean and repair itself. Think back to a time when you were sick or forced to be in bed for long stretches of time. Did your body feel unusually sore and stiff even though you didn't workout?

Your body needs movement in order to stay healthy. Both liver tossing and shaking exercise can be done throughout the day. 2-5 minutes is a good starting point. The more times you can do it throughout the day, the better.

These next exercises are based on delivering the desired stress response we spoke about at the beginning of this section. Remember, the reason they bring benefits to you is because they are uncomfortable. If you can reach the recommended time for each stimulus, you will reap the benefits that come along with them.

Start small in the beginning. You can always do more next time, but you can't do less. It's the same principle discussed earlier. Don't try to run a marathon if you haven't run 3km before. Start slowly and build yourself up.

Heat Exposure

Heat exposure is perhaps one of the more fun and easy ways to trigger fat loss along with eustress. There are even benefits to longevity, cardiovascular health, neurodegenerative protection, toxin elimination, and mood enhancements.

A study from Finland that followed 2,300 men for 20 years shows some incredible evidence for the benefits of heat exposure coming from the use of a sauna. The study found that men who used a Finish dry sauna for 19 minutes at 80-100 degrees Celsius had a drastic reduction in 3 key areas of health.

Men who used the sauna under these conditions 4-7 times

a week saw a 40% reduction in all-cause mortality. This means they were 40% less likely to die from anything compared to those that went once a week. They were 50% less likely to die from cardiovascular problems and 65% less likely to develop Alzheimer's and dementia. These are pretty incredible results considering you're just sitting there.

Another benefit of heat is that it helps stimulate heat shock proteins. These specific proteins help slow down muscle wasting as you age. They also help prevent protein aggregation, which may be why saunas aid in reducing neurodegenerative diseases and cardiovascular problems.

The benefits of the sauna may partially come from their ability to mimic moderate physical activity. The sauna is tricking your body into producing similar health responses as working out at a moderate pace. Your heart rate increases above resting and can even reach 150 beats per minute, as if you were running. Sweat is stimulated to help cool you down during this process.

This stimulation helps to train your heart, arteries, and veins in a similar way as exercise would. Improvements in your arteries can be seen as well as an improvement in blood pressure. It also moves a lot of blood through your muscles and joints, delivering nutrients and removing waste, which helps with recovery and pain.

One of my first experiences with a sauna was when I was 18 years old. I found myself in a sauna with a girl I happened to like quite a bit. We pushed ourselves to complete 15 minutes. As soon as I stepped out, I noticed that my back was riddled with giant pimples. My body had detoxed years of pizza, donuts, chips, and any fast food chain you can think of in a matter of minutes.

I had found out the hard way that the skin is a major detox organ. The sauna had mobilized so many of my toxins and pushed them into my back for excretion. For the next week I was trying my best to hide this but it was near impossible. The sauna is an excellent way to boost your detox systems, especially if you experience skin or digestive issues.

Sweating is a natural way for your body to rid itself of toxins. If you tend to have sweat that smells, that can be toxins trying to clear out of your body. Heavy metals and even BPA can be released while in the sauna. Toxins that your body hasn't been able to process internally are now being released through your skin so your body doesn't have to deal with it internally.

Sauna use can even have a strong effect on your mood from its impact on brain neurochemistry. A chemical known as dynorphin (opposite of endorphins) is released in your brain to signal distress or pain. You've probably heard of endorphins, which produce positive feelings and emotions.

When you initially enter a sauna, you feel content. As time goes on, you get a sense of discomfort and eventually can't tolerate being there anymore. As a meditative practice, this is when the sauna begins to show its strength. When the dynorphin builds up, it becomes much harder to think about anything other than the present moment. Equanimity becomes important. This is a natural survival mechanism to help you focus on getting out of pain and stress. It also has a huge benefit to your mood.

As you become continually more and more uncomfortable from prolonged heat exposure, dynorphin builds up to signal you to leave. When you resist the urge to leave and go into discomfort, your brain increases the receptors for endorphins, making you more sensitive to them. This means that you need less endorphins to give you good feelings.

If you don't have much experience with saunas, don't be a hero the first time you go. Make sure you are well hydrated as this will greatly impact your ability to stay in the sauna. You want to push past your comfort level but listen to your body as well. Start with less time and gradually build up. 19 minutes seems to be the sweet spot to build towards. Make sure to shower afterwards in order to remove the sweat and toxins.

Cold Exposure

The benefits of cold exposure can be experienced and seen on many levels. A commitment to exposing your body to cold for short bursts will boost your metabolism, drastically enhance your mood, improve your immune system, decrease inflammation, induce a meditative state, and improve your circulatory system.

The increase in metabolism from cold exposure is due to the added stimulation of thermogenesis. This is the creation of heat through metabolism. There are two main mechanisms to this. As you become colder, your body naturally wants to heat itself up which costs calories. It does so by causing your muscles to contract, making you shiver to generate heat. This is similar to the way you would feel warm after you started exercising.

The other way to increase thermogenesis is through the use of BAT (brown adipose tissue). As discussed earlier, BAT is a highly metabolic type of fat that burns calories from white (regular) fat tissue to generate heat. When you practice consistent cold exposure, you help increase your body's natural stores of BAT which in turn helps you burn even more white fat.

Cold exposure also helps to keep you healthy and on track with your weight loss by boosting your immunity. Repeated exposure can help signal the creation of more white blood cells, which help fight harmful invaders. If you can avoid getting sick, it will be much easier to stick to your weight loss goals.

This type of training also helps to generate cold shock proteins. Much like heat shock proteins, they help slow down neurodegenerative aging of the synapses in your brain. Cold therapy can aid with protecting your brain function as you age so you stay sharp and highly capable of taking care of yourself.

Using cold exposure is like cheating when it comes to concentration and meditation. Unlike sitting still and forcing yourself to meditate, plunging into cold water immediately grabs your attention. Cold exposure doesn't have to be in an ice bath. It can be a cold shower, a dip in the snow, or just standing out in the cold weather.

When you go into the cold, your body releases norepinephrine as a hormone to help you retain heat. Norepinephrine helps constrict your peripheral veins and arteries in order to shuttle warm blood to your organs. This is a natural defensive response that, when triggered, acts as a powerful hormedic and eustress stimulus.

Inflammation is a key factor in aging and is involved in many disease processes. When norepinephrine is stimulated with cold training, it can help inhibit something known as TNF-alpha, which normally produces inflammatory cytokines. This systematic reduction of inflammation also acts as a pain reliever since inflammation tends to cause pain.

During cold exposure, norepinephrine is also released as a neurotransmitter in your brain. This is what's responsible for you entering a fight or flight mode. It causes you to focus deeply into the moment and forget about the troubles of the past and future. It truly pulls you into the moment like few other things can because your survival is at stake with these conditions.

You have about 100,000 km of blood vessels in your body. Cold exposure forces the contraction of the vessels which in effect helps to train your circulatory system. Much like your visible muscles, these vessels have muscles that want to be trained in order to maintain their strength and flexibility. Having nimble blood vessels helps with blood pressure regulation and heart health.

As a meditative practice, cold exposure teaches you equanimity and allows you to practice being in fight or flight under your terms. Within seconds of cold exposure, your body demands you move out of that environment because it doesn't want to deal with the shock of the cold. Through your willpower, you can sit in the metaphorical eye of the storm and learn to remain calm when your body is screaming at you.

A mere 30 seconds is all it takes to start a cascade of beneficial effects. 2 minutes is the ideal time to build up to in order to trigger most benefits you will receive from cold exposure. Anything beyond that is not necessary unless you're planning on doing an event that requires extreme cold exposure. Too much cold exposure can have a negative impact.

Every time I've overdone a cold exposure, I've ended up making myself sick. If you're outdoors swimming in cold water, make sure to put clothes on ASAP after. You want to avoid getting cut up by the wind on your bare skin. You can easily overdose on cold exposure and should start off with about 30 seconds if you're not used to it.

Cold exposure can be done daily to help you with weight loss along with the benefits just discussed. These are by no means limits to the benefits of cold exposure. Once again, start with 30 seconds of either a cold shower, ice bath, or cold weather exposure. Build yourself up to 2 minutes daily and you will reap most of the benefits from this therapy.

Bridge the Gap

A summary of the techniques mentioned in this section are provided below. Pick and choose the ones that resonate best with you. It's better to have a few practices that you can develop versus switching between too many and building skill with none.

Breathing

    1. Nose Breathing

    2. Diaphragm Activation

    3. 4 in, 2 out

    4. 4x4 Breathe

    5. Slow Breathing

    6. Breath Holds (Full and Empty Lungs)

    7. Walking Breath Holds

    8. Othership App

Meditation

    1. Contemplative Meditation

        a. Concentration

        b. Sensory Clarity

        c. Equanimity

    2. Physical Acts of Meditation

        a. Liver Qi Tossing

        b. Shaking

        c. Heat Exposure

        d. Cold Exposure

BONUS: LOOK YOUNGER, ADD SEX APPEAL, & ACCELERATE YOUR RESULTS

" The better developed and balanced his muscular system, the healthier and better functioning will be his mind"
- Eugen Sandow

I cannot write a book about holistic weight loss without paying tribute to the importance of exercising. If you don't want to workout to lose weight you don't need to. You can put this book down right now. However, if you want to accelerate your weight loss, look younger, increase your strength, reduce joint and muscle pain, and improve the overall quality of your life, I highly suggest you read onwards.

Working out has massive benefits for your hormones and will accelerate the effects of everything you have read thus far. Working out a few times a week significantly improves your mood, your waistline, your sleep, your diet, flexibility, and your stress levels. This final Bonus section will cover all the benefits of adding exercise to your weight loss and overall lifestyle plan.

It's important to be specific when I use the word "exercise". As stated earlier, I'm not a fan of training just for the sake of getting your heart rate up, sweating, and "working hard". When I write about working out, it's with the express focus of qualitatively and quantitatively training your strength in order to maintain or even build muscle mass as you lose fat.

When you lose weight without proper strength training, you are inadvertently losing muscle mass alongside the fat. Muscle is a highly metabolic tissue that contributes greatly to your daily calorie consumption and what is known as RMR (resting metabolic rate). RMR is the amount of calories your body burns to perform life-sustaining functions. RMR accounts for 60-75% of daily energy expenditure. Anything above just resting in bed all day will increase the amount of calories you burn.

Why Muscle Matters

You're about to read some examples of fat loss calculations using calories. Although I'm not a huge fan of counting calories, I've included them here because I believe it will demonstrate the power of strength training when it comes to weight loss. As one loses weight, their metabolism tends to decrease as well. Strength training is the secret sauce to maintaining your metabolism so you can still enjoy food without having to cut calories on purpose.

Someone who has more muscle mass will tend to have a higher metabolism. 1 pound of lean muscle mass burns approximately 6 calories per day while 1 pound of fat will burn approximately 2 calories. For every additional pound of muscle weight compared to fat weight, you are burning 4 extra calories while resting. If two people weigh the same amount but one person has more muscle mass, their metabolism will be higher.

Let's compare two men who both weigh 200lbs. Imagine we take them through a DEXA scan, which is a method of measuring a person's body, that allows us to see how much muscle mass vs fat mass each individual has. One man has 100lbs muscles while the other man is much leaner and has 150lbs of muscle. The leaner man will have 50lbs multiplied by an extra 4 calories per day meaning that he can burn an additional 200 calories a day while simply resting.

Over a one month period, that adds up to a significant difference. Burning an additional 200 calories a day for 30 days leads to 6,000 calories being spent while resting and before he even does anything else. There are approximately 3,500 calories stored in 1 pound of fat. That means the leaner man is burning almost 2lbs worth of extra calories per month. Over the course of a year, that equates to 73,000 calories or an extra 20lbs of potential fat. These extra calories can be the difference in you sustaining your weight loss if you indulge in a cheat meal from time to time.

It gets better than that. The reality is that the more muscular man will also be working out which adds to his energy expenditure. Doing a 1-hour workout can burn anywhere from 400-800 calories depending on your size and intensity. Building strength and muscle allows you to burn additional calories while in the gym but also while you're at rest. Compared to someone that does not exercise, the ability to shed extra fat is undeniable.

If two people weigh the same amount but one of them is much leaner than the other, the leaner person can eat more food during the day and still maintain or even lose weight. Since they train in the gym, burn more calories while at rest, and induce a lower insulin response when they eat (more about this soon), they are able to maintain a higher metabolism. This means they can enjoy more of the foods they want without the negative side effects that someone who wasn't training would experience.

Let's make this more relevant for you using some hypothetical numbers. Imagine your initial starting weight was 250lbs with 150lbs of that being lean muscle mass (anything other than fat), you would have a body fat percentage of 40%. If you got down to a weight of 150lbs and didn't engage in strength training, we can estimate that you lost 50lbs of fat in the process and 50lbs of muscle. You would now be down to a body fat percentage of 33.3%.

If you were able to achieve the same amount of weight loss but you chose to use strength training to get there, something magical would happen. Instead of losing the hypothetical 50lbs of muscle, you could have lost 80lbs of fat and only 20lbs of muscle, leaving you at a sexy and toned 13% body fat. You would also have an additional 30lbs of muscle burning an extra 120 calories per day.

Let's break this down into practical numbers. At 150lbs, over the course of a 1 month, you would burn an additional 120 calories per day, multiplied by 30 days, giving you 3,600 calories. During the same month, let's assume you did just 3, one hour workouts per week, burning 500 calories. That's an extra 1,500 calories per week. All together that's 3,600 + 6000 calories giving you 9,600 additional calories. That's an extra 2.75lbs lost compared to someone who didn't train.

There is, however, something I've yet to mention about this equation. For people who want to lose weight and are already lean, let's say 15% body fat or below, it is harder to lose fat and build muscle simultaneously. For someone who has a higher body fat percentage of 20% or more, it is possible for them to maintain most of their muscle mass or even build some muscle while losing fat. As you get leaner, it becomes more difficult to build muscle while losing fat at the same time.

Although it is exciting to see how much more calories you burn when maintaining muscle, one simple fact cannot be overlooked. As you lose weight, you are losing fat and therefore, you are losing the energy expenditure you would have had from that fat. If you lose 80lbs of fat, you lose that additional 160 calories per day (80lbs of fat multiplied by 2 calories burned per day). This is why it's so important to use strength training to burn calories while in the gym but also to maintain muscle mass in order to keep your metabolism up.

If all of that was too theoretical or difficult to grasp, you can go to Radoslav.ca/StengthTraining. There is a video of me explaining all of this as well using a white board and writing everything out in a simple format.

Strength Training is Optimal

The benefits of strength training become even clearer when we compare all this to the alternative of crash diets. Focusing on calorie deficits and high heart rate workouts that don't build strength or muscle results in the opposite. Less muscle and a lower metabolism. Without proper stimulation for strength and hypertrophy (a fancy word for building muscle), you lose out on the benefits described above and move in the opposite direction.

High heart rate cardio workouts tend to train endurance. Endurance training leads to a destruction of muscle mass and a ramping up of your appetite. Your body adapts to the stimulus you put on it. Since muscle is energy consumptive and since the stimulation you're giving your body is for endurance, it moves towards those adaptations. Reducing muscle mass aids in endurance. Without going into the physiology of why this happens, simply looking at the difference in the physique of a marathon runner and a sprinter makes my point. We can also consider professional fighters as an example. Those in lower weight classes have much better endurance and speed compared to those in higher weight classes.

If you have experienced this in the past you may now realize why this type of training and calorie deficit diets don't work. Without muscle and strength preservation while losing weight, you decrease your metabolism significantly. In order to maintain weight loss along with your sanity, strength training is highly advisable.

Not only would you have a higher metabolism, which is also aided from additional caloric expenditure from training, but your body would look more toned and muscular. After all, your body is represented in how you look and how your clothes fit and not by an artificial number on a scale. If you want an athletic and lean look, you need to train for it. Your weight doesn't always translate to the look and feel you want from your body.

Having gone through all that, I need you to understand that those calories and numbers are not perfect. They are there for demonstration purposes so you understand the underlying process. In reality, it isn't as clean as I have laid it out but the principles apply.

Benefits Beyond Fat-Loss

There are many added benefits to training that go beyond calorie expenditure. Living pain free and aging with strength is critical to your enjoyment of life. Being in chronic pain because your muscles, bones, and joints are too weak due to neglect should not be your goal. Training also keeps your heart, lungs, and digestion healthy.

Having real world strength that allows you to play, enjoy your hobbies, be outdoors with friends, family, and your kids is far more important than just hitting the number on the scale. Being able to indulge in good food from time to time is also important. Using methods like strength training to balance this out significantly improves your chances of success and compliance with your commitments.

Muscle is also beneficial from a vanity point of view. As a man, it feels good to have powerful arms, wide shoulders, and a broad chest. As a woman, it feels nice to have a firm butt that perks up in jeans, yoga pants, and even a bikini. Strong sexy legs and a toned waist with a few abs poking through isn't all that bad either.

The mental, emotional, and spiritual components of training are also extremely powerful. This goes back to my analogy of treating your body like a dog. When you exercise, it's the equivalent of taking your dog out for an hour-long walk. When you return home, your dog is calm, happy, and quiet. Exercise is also known to help with sadness and depression by boosting one's mood.

If you're over the age of 50, strength training is extremely important. Muscle mass fades with age and becomes more difficult to build and maintain the older you are. Bones become brittle and osteoporosis becomes a reality. Strength training will help maintain your muscles as you age while also increasing your bone density.

Those of you who are 70+ years or approaching it really need to pay attention to training. The threat of falling has become a reality as 4.5% of 70 year olds die from falling. I'm not talking about falling down stairs, I mean falling from the height you are while just standing. That's a 1/20 chance of dying from a simple and preventable accident. Quality of life is also diminished as recovering from a hip injury or fracture takes more time. Having the strength, balance, coordination and reflexes to catch yourself is critical. All of these can be greatly enhanced with a workout routine.

Overall strength is a key indicator of health as one ages. The strength of one's grip can be used to measure this and to predict all causes mortality, bone density, depression, cognitive impairment and even sleep. The stronger your grip, the less likely you are to be impacted by these negative side effects.

Regardless of what reasons motivate you to train, be they superficial or intrinsic, the benefits speak for themselves. We will now briefly discuss the hormonal impact of strength training and maintaining muscle. I will also put an end to the myth that crunches are the best way to trim your midsection and get abs once and for all.

Hormonal Benefits

As you lose weight you will improve your insulin sensitivity. The more muscle you have in your body relative to fat, the more insulin sensitive you become. Someone who is at a lean 10% body fat requires less insulin when they eat a meal compared to someone who is at 20% or 30% body fat. Working out can also increase your insulin sensitivity.

Training consumes some of your stored muscle glycogen. Emptying the muscles of their glycogen will cause insulin to store calories into the muscles before storing them as fat. Therefore, workouts are a great tool to reduce the impact of a meal. When you eat, if your muscle glycogen store has been depleted, energy will be preferentially stored there before it goes to fat. If you never train and never empty your muscle glycogen, food will always go directly to fat storage.

Working out also benefits two other key hormones in your body, those being testosterone and human growth hormones. Both are crucial for the growth and repair of your body. If you have low testosterone, whether you're a male or female, it's going to impact your ability to lose weight, maintain muscle, and even your mood. Human growth hormones will also impact these.

Testosterone deficiency can show up in many ways. Symptoms of fatigue, poor mood, anemia and reduced sex drive along with excess fat storage are signs of low testosterone. As we age, testosterone tends to decline, making weight loss more challenging. The good news is that with lifestyle adjustments and strength training, you can improve your testosterone levels.

If you're deficient in human growth hormone production, similar problems occur. Adults who are below normal levels of growth hormone tend to have more body fat (especially in the waist). They also tend to suffer from fatigue, anxiety, depression, and experience a decrease in sexual function. Training can help restore this imbalance when combined with all the lifestyle factors mentioned in this book.

If you are over the age of 50 and feel as though you are slowing down, you might want to consider hormone therapy from a qualified profession. You can get your blood tested to see if you have deficiencies in your hormones. This will be different for males and females which is why it's crucial to go to someone knowledgeable and reputable.

As we age, our bodies stop functioning to their previous abilities. A large part of that is hormone related. Once your levels are measured, you can use the hormones to bring your levels back to normal. Getting this addressed can enhance your fat loss, mood, and overall health. Although I believe many things can be solved with lifestyle changes, if you feel like you're doing a lot of things right and still not seeing results, this could be worth researching for yourself.

Training to Maximize Fat-Loss

Muscle and strength preservation is of utmost importance when it comes to working out for fat-loss. In order to achieve this, there are a few rules we need to follow. The more you can adhere to these, the better your fat-loss results will be and the better your body composition will be.

Focusing on full-body workouts is important when fat loss is your main goal. Although there are many great ways to structure a program, I've found that full body training is usually best for most beginners and even those with some moderate experience is best. The more muscles we can engage during the workout, the more calories we can burn. We are also sending a bigger signal to our body which in turn helps release testosterone and growth hormones.

Imagine two possibilities when it comes to training. Focusing on one body part versus focusing on the whole body. If you were to just train your arms, chest, or back during a single workout, you're only accessing a limited amount of the muscles in your body. When you do a full body workout, you're now stimulating and demanding so much more from your body.

Compound exercises are the best solution for this. A compound exercise involves multiple joints and muscles in the body, whereas something like an isolation exercise focuses on one joint or specific muscle. A bodyweight squat is an example of a compound exercise. It involves your butt, thighs, and calves. A bicep curl would be an example of an isolation exercise. Having a workout routine that is predominately made up of compound exercises that target the entire body each time will likely be the best option for you.

There is a major myth that I'm going to debunk right now. Doing exercises like crunches and sit ups will not burn the fat around your midsection. Dedicating 30-60 minutes to training your abs is not a good approach to removing belly fat. Unlike glycogen that's stored in your muscles, fat is burned from the entire body and not one localized point. Therefore, you're better off spending your time engaging as many muscles as possible instead of initiating one small group of muscles.

The other reason I don't like exercises like crunches is because they destroy your posture and can lead to neck and lower back pain. I'm going to go out on a limb here and assume you spend a good chunk of your day looking at a computer, cell phone, or tv screen. Heck, even if you're reading books all day, you could be suffering from this. By doing so, you are likely spending a large portion of your day in a crunched position with poor posture.

If you're already spending 10 hours a day in this position, the last thing you want to do is spend your workouts reinforcing this bad position. I've watched enough "core" workout videos to see that this is an unfortunate reality of bad program design and people are suffering from it. A good workout is needed to address posture and build up back muscles that are often neglected and weakened from poor posture.

A good program will emphasize posture in every movement. Without good posture, your joints, especially in your spine, come out of alignment and take unnecessary wear and tear. When posture is addressed, not only are injuries less likely but you are also more likely to be adhering to the following principles.

Slow and controlled movements are the foundations of any quality fat-loss, strength training, and muscle building program. This is one of the main reasons I don't promote high intensity workouts for beginners. When you're learning (or relearning) to train properly, you need to make slow, deliberate, and controlled movements. This ensures that your muscles take the tension and not your joints.

The slower you are, the easier it will be to produce good biomechanics. You know this to be true. The faster you try to do something, the less accurate you become at it. I'm not saying you need to move like a turtle but you do need to move with grace and intention. This leads me to the next crucial variable to producing results.

The ability to connect to your muscles and put your full attention there is a beautiful thing. It helps ensure that you're using muscles you want and will help keep the tension there instead of in your joints. Connecting to your muscles and feeling it work is a meditation practice in itself. To truly connect and be there to experience your body putting out a high level of intensity and effort is beautiful.

With all this being said, we can finally discuss intensity during an exercise and during a workout. Again, high intensity for the sake of sweating and raising your heart rate will have most beginners putting a tremendous load through their joints instead of their muscles. You want to focus the intensity into your muscles. This will help improve your strength, build muscle and prevent injury.

There are many other factors such as reps, sets, rest time, total volume, and exercise selection that go into making a program. If you're interested in a holistic fat loss program, go to my website, www.Radoslav.ca/FatLossWorkouts and you'll be taken to a program I designed to go specifically with this book.

Everything in this book will work in perfect harmony with the training provided there. It's 4 months of full body exercise, taught by me, to help ensure you burn fat. Training should get you results while being something enjoyable and sustainable. I have put my heart, soul, and knowledge into that program to make sure you succeed.

The workouts last from 20-40 minutes depending on how you do them. There is no-equipment required and you can do it from the comfort of your own home. The workouts are designed with beginners in mind and those who are trying to lose weight. Even if you have a good foundation in training, you will find this program valuable. There are 71 unique exercises that come together in 3 phases.

Detailed explanations and modifications are provided for every exercise and workout. There is simply no room left for confusion. Ready-Made-Logs are provided for you to track your progress. If you want a program that's designed with you in mind and in harmony with the recommendations in this book, I invite you to check it out.

The End of This Book, The Start of Your Journey

You are now equipped to make the necessary changes to your habits to transform your life. I wish you all the best on your journey and may this book serve as a guide to help you keep moving forward. If you found it useful, please share the knowledge. Having you become a beacon of health is one of my goals.

Lead by example in your life and people will follow. If there is a significant person who you wish to help, the greatest way to impact them is to succeed on your own journey. No one wants to be told what to do. They want to see what's possible. Once they've seen your transformation and are ready for guidance, they will ask you for it.

If you enjoyed reading this book and found it helpful, consider leaving an honest review where you purchased it so that you can help others make the decision to get the book. It doesn't have to be a long review and even just hitting the stars goes a long way. I sincerely hope this book adds value to your life and wish you all the best on your journey. If you want to keep up with my latest health tips, you can follow me here:

TikTok = RadRadoslav

Instagram = RadRadoslav

Youtube = Radoslav Detchev

Printed in Great Britain
by Amazon

82633288R10108